Birth Days: Inspiring Stories of Healing and Transformation in Childbirth
Mindy R. Levy

Producer & International Distributor
eBookPro Publishing
www.ebook-pro.com

Birth Days: Inspiring Stories of Healing and Transformation in Childbirth
Mindy R. Levy

Copyright © 2022 Mindy R. Levy

All rights reserved; No parts of this book may be reproduced or transmitted in any form or by any means, electronic or mechanical, including photocopying, recording, taping, or by any information retrieval system, without the permission, in writing, of the author.

Illustrations by Miri Sgan-Cohen

Contact: mindwife@gmail.com
ISBN 9798218371418

Birth Days

Inspiring Stories of Healing and Transformation in Childbirth

Mindy R. Levy

Contents

Deganit	8
Introduction: Where Trauma Meets Birth	11
My Births – The Bad, The Good and The Ugly	17
Becoming Mindwife	27
An Excerpt from my Thesis Journal	30
Journal Entry: Searching for Connections	33
Journal Entry: What I Have Learned about Birth by Studying about Trauma	36
Learning to Listen to Women in the Delivery Room	45
Only Six Centimeters	45
More Luck than Brains	47
Journal Entry: Honoring Intuition	49
Too Busy to Birth	51
Natural Twins	53
Nila	55
The Truck and the Motorcycle	60
Not According to the Plan	62
Just Like Her Cat	65
Labor Positions	68
Knee-Chest Position	69
On All Fours	71
Standing Up for Herself	73
Closed Legs	76

Women are Capable of Anything – Births at Home	**79**
Saying Yes from Now On	80
A Single Mom and a New Pool	86
Pushing on One Leg	90
Doing it her Way	95
Just A Few Hours Later	99
Backing Up and Backing Off	102
Surprise!	107
Giving Birth in Peace	111
Not Here to Make Friends	119
A Breath of Fresh Air	128
Births at Agoola	**133**
Journal Entry, July 7, 2004	134
The Vision and the Construction	136
The Premier	138
Michal's Two Births	142
Pizza in the Oven	150
Star-Crossed Mothers	154
Closing and Opening the Doors	160
Ayelet's Three Births	162
Regaining Faith in Her Body	162
A Premie in Agoola	164
Three is a Lucky Number	166
The Birth of a Baby, a Mother, and a Grandmother	170
Face to Face	174

Finding a Better Way – The VBAC Heroines	**179**
With Her Head Held High – Ma'ayan	181
Good Enough – Shlomit	185
Finally Feeling the Urge	188
VBAC, Hey!!!	196
Noa's Cesarean Party	203
Inspiring Work with Abuse Survivors	**211**
The Births of Aya and Noga	212
More Safety, Less Intimacy – Anat	223
Taking a Deep Breath – Ayelet	232
Riding the Horse – Efi	238
Orly The Lioness	247
Winding Down – The End of an Era	**259**
One Last Story – Gal's #3, My #444	261
Epilogue – Dear Duggi	**265**
It's a Boy! (Obviously) 7 September 2010	267
How to Survive an Israeli Hospital – 8 September 2010	269
Call the Midwife – On Home Births in the North of Israel	274
3 March 2013	274
Frequently Asked Questions	277
It's a Boy! (again) Home Birth No.2 11 March 2016	280
A Girl? You Can't Be Serious 12 May 2018	282
My Eulogy at Deganit's Funeral	**286**
Acknowledgments	**288**
References	**290**

Dedicated to Deganit

Deganit, a dear friend and client passed away prematurely at age 40. She left behind five wonderful children, an adoring husband, two unpublished books and a lot of stories. As a lover of storytelling, she told me many times that I must put my stories down on paper and write a book. She suggested that I call it my "Mindoirs." She thought I could teach a lot about birth to a lot of women, and she was willing to help me get started. She even offered to sit with me and listen to my stories, record the conversations and then help me to put them into written form.

We never got around to it. We both thought that we had all the time in the world. And then she died. It took over a week before I realized that in addition to losing her as a friend and as a client, I had also lost her as my writing associate. My first impulse was to say to myself, "OK, I get the message. This was not meant to be." After a few weeks, I realized that the opposite was the case. Now that she had left her body, she had lots of free time to listen and we could do this together. We will forever be each other's inspirations, sounding boards, fan clubs and creative associates.

I imagined the day would come when I would be ripe enough to write my book. It would be in a wooden cabin by a lake. I would be alone with no telephone, television or other distractions. I would have endless cups of tea or coffee by my side, as I poured my heart out onto the keys of my laptop. But here I am – no lake, no cabin. My husband is in the next room, my telephone is on the table near me

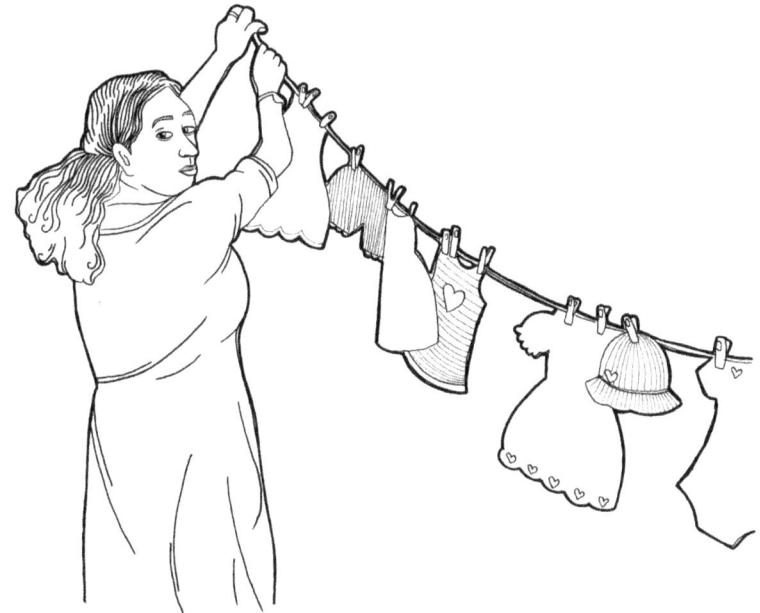

and lunch is simmering on the stove. I am alone with my laptop, just me and the words that are making their way out of my mind into my fingers on the keys and onto the screen. Not a cup of tea in sight.

Yet, Deganit is with me, cheering me on and feeling proud of me. The time has come to open my journals, make sense of my experiences and see what I can pass on to others. Deganit is by my side, and she is my muse.

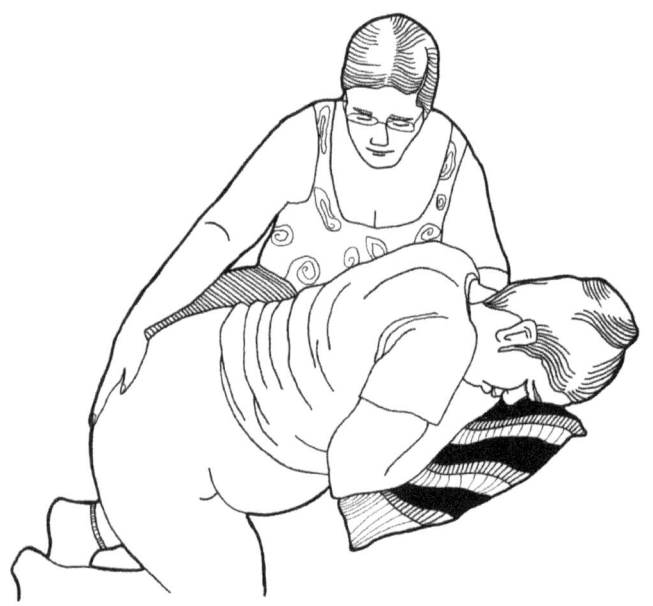

Introduction: Where Trauma Meets Birth

Today I understand and know that there is a clear and important connection between birth and trauma. It wasn't always so obvious to me, but over time, it has evolved into being the focus of my energies, my work, my research, my writings and my teachings. I firmly believe that in that place where trauma and maternity meet, healing can happen. Writing this book and exploring the evolution of this belief have enabled me to reconnect with my journey through the land where trauma meets birth.

In the delivery room, working as a new and enthusiastic midwife, I often noticed women whose reactions to labor seemed out of the ordinary. They seemed to be suffering too much and not at all in proportion to the physical strength of their uterine contractions. Sometimes these women seemed to be in another world, not present in their bodies and certainly not present in the here and now. Sometimes they screamed. Sometimes they cried incessantly. Sometimes they hyperventilated. Sometimes they hid under the bed sheets and avoided eye contact. Sometimes they relentlessly asked one question after another, trying to gain some sense of control over the situation by gathering information from as many different sources as possible. They managed to irritate everyone involved and acquired colorful and derogative labels from the staff in the process.

Some women were okay during the first stage of labor while their cervix was dilating but became agitated when it came time to push.

They would swallow the baby's head back into the vagina with each contraction while making pushing sounds and feigning pushing efforts. They had long second stages, swollen labia and were often threatened with vacuum deliveries. As time became the critical factor, more members of the medical team would enter the room, encouraging, sometimes shouting, holding the woman's legs open, tugging on her perineum, pressing on her abdomen and doing whatever was deemed necessary to get the baby out. When the babies were born the mothers were distanced, dazed, exhausted and disconnected. These babies started life alone in a plastic bassinet while their mothers needed time to gather themselves back together, figure out if the battle was over and check if it was safe to come back to the here and now.

Other women were okay when they got to the second stage, the pushing-the-baby-out stage but had much more difficulty getting through the first stage while coping with the pain of cervical dilation. They seemed to be in pain even during the pauses in between the contractions. They seemed tormented and terrorized, triggered by something unrelated to the physiological process. Some women didn't want to hold their babies after they were born. Many didn't want to put them to the breast. They just wanted to rest and be left alone.

Some women never went into labor even after going to 42 weeks and more. What was that about? What was going on with those women hormonally that their bodies couldn't let go of the pregnancy? What made them so afraid that their bodies held on for dear life to the fruit they had produced and couldn't allow it to fall from the tree?

I began to talk with my fellow midwives about trauma because these women seemed traumatized to me, even though I knew very little about trauma at the time. I earned a reputation in the delivery room and was labeled as being obsessed with the notion of trauma playing a critical role in the birth experience. For me, it was a fact. I began to understand that something about the experience of birth causes traumas to resurface. They appear like thieves in the night; they steal away the flow of the birth process, making it much longer and more painful and turning pain into suffering.

The brighter side of this understanding was that birth is also a golden opportunity for healing. Because of its power, significance, and emotional and physical impact, a positive, empowering birth experience can change a woman forever. A vaginal birth after a Cesarean can put a woman back on track to believing in herself and her body. For a woman who suffers from vaginismus experiencing her baby coming through her vagina can forever change the story that her vagina tells about itself. For a woman who had a long, excruciating first birth, a quick, easy second birth can change the way she sees herself. For a woman with a history of sexual abuse, a birth in an atmosphere of privacy, respect, control, information and compassion can change the way she relates to her body and the world.

After I left the hospital and started doing home births, I had a lot more time to get to know the pregnant women I was delivering. We invested hours in getting to know one another, building trust and confidence and creating a safe space. More and more women with traumatic histories found their way to my clinic. During the fifteen years I worked as a home birth midwife, I delivered the babies of over a hundred survivors of sexual violence. I accompanied numerous emergency C-section survivors through the challenge of making peace with their stories and achieving a normal, natural, empowering vaginal birth. Women with other traumas came to my clinic, and gradually I gained more experience and knowledge from each woman, each pregnancy and each birth.

I went to Africa and worked with midwives there. I sat with them and listened to their stories. When I felt comfortable enough, I initiated discussions on the topic of trauma and its connection with birth. These women were more than willing to share their stories, their hardships and frustrations, their traumas and the sources of their healing.

Some were unique to their personal experience, their culture and their environment; some were universal to birthing women everywhere.

I learned that the possibilities for healing are as present and significant as the dangers of retraumatization during birth everywhere on the planet. What happens is not the arbitrary result of a coin flip. There will always be circumstances beyond our control; that is a fact. But healing is a choice we make, and the journey begins when we choose to pursue a corrective experience, to look for a better way, to search for a different place, to learn a new approach, to find the right support people and to dig deeper inside ourselves to discover what is truly right for each one of us.

This book is about my journey in becoming a trauma-sensitive midwife. It is about how I learned to listen and to learn midwifery from the women I had the honor and the privilege to accompany on their journeys. It is about making mistakes and learning from them. It is about the potential for healing that is buried within each and every one of us. It is about giving life and being born.

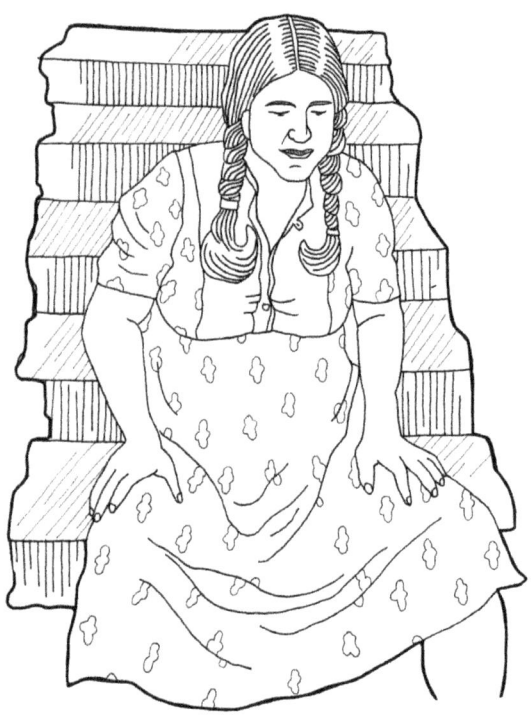

My Births – The Bad, The Good and The Ugly

In exploring the connection between trauma and birth, I am compelled to start by exploring my own birth experiences. Maybe my attitude and observations have been colored by my own attitude toward pregnancy and my own births. Did I become super sensitive to this issue because of my personal birth history?

For as long as I can remember, I was fascinated with pregnancy and birth. As a young girl, I would stop and stare at pregnant women on the street wondering about what was happening inside their bodies. That fascination remains with me even today when I pause and focus my gaze on a woman's body that contains another complete human being inside it. I wonder how all this could even be possible. Pregnancy is a remarkable process, and the birth of every healthy baby is truly a miracle. I have never lost that sense of wonder and amazement about birth. It still knocks me off my feet every time I witness it.

I enjoyed being pregnant. I felt special, different, engaged in a big long-term project, a challenge, an act of creation.

At times I felt like I had been taken over by aliens like my body was out of my control and had a mind of its own. This neither scared nor upset me, and I loved feeling my babies move inside my belly. Pregnancy was also a lesson in letting go, mostly letting go of control.

I planned for a natural birth. I wasn't quite sure what that meant, but I had a deep, personal understanding that drugs and giving birth should not go together. I was inspired by the women in Ina May Gaskin's book,

Spiritual Midwifery, which I read early on in my pregnancy. I believed in myself and my body.

I was young and healthy when I had my babies. The three of them were born within less than four years. I gave birth in three different hospitals and had three very different birth experiences. They contained traumatic elements, but I doubt the difficult parts would be classified as traumatic by anyone other than me.

My first son Udi was born in Carmel Hospital in Haifa when I was 25 years old. I prepared for a natural birth by attending childbirth preparation classes together with my husband Avner and was ready for a good experience. I was young, excited, enthusiastic and in love. I am American and have Polish and Russian genes. I was curious to discover what combination my lily-white chromosomes and my husband's dark, curly-haired Yemenite ones would produce. It was before the age of ultrasound scans, and we didn't know the sex of the fetus in my womb. Avner was hoping for a girl, and I was sure that it was a boy.

I was 39 weeks pregnant, exactly a week before my due date. My contractions started at about 3 am. I woke Avner up at about 5:30, and we left the house for the hospital around 6:30. We had moved from Beer Sheva to Tivon four days earlier, and our moving and cleaning helpers were still asleep on the couches. One of them lived in Haifa, so we woke him up to offer him a ride home. Barry thought we were joking and went back to sleep. We arrived at the hospital together with the midwives working the morning shift. I was told that I was four centimeters dilated. I received a shave, an enema, a shower and a hospital dressing gown and I was hooked up to a fetal monitor.

My memory is fuzzy. I remember that Avner was allowed to be with me in the only room where husbands were permitted entry because we had done the childbirth preparation class together. I remember being connected to the monitor the entire time until the baby was born. I remember lying on my left side and not being permitted to move, turn around or change positions because otherwise the monitor wouldn't work. I had a backache that I will never forget as long as I live, and I was unable to relieve the pain in any way. It felt like a knife was cutting through my back, relentlessly digging and causing unbearable pain which got worse as time went on. I remember lying on a bed so high and narrow, with a mattress so thin, that it was almost impossible to turn around even if the monitor cords would have been long enough to allow me to do so.

I breathed through the contractions and held onto Avner's big, strong hand for dear life. We were both nervous and excited, and our reaction was to laugh, mostly during the breaks in between contractions. Everything seemed funny even though the pain of the contractions was very real. The movement of my belly laughter was broadcasted through the microphone of the monitor and also appeared on the monitor strip. This frivolous behavior was frowned upon by the staff, and we wondered whether or not they would kick us out and send us home because of the ruckus we were creating.

During each contraction, I crunched Avner's hand mercilessly as the pain became more intense. He knew exactly how much pain I was experiencing because his poor hand caught the brunt of it. As the contractions became more intense, I felt myself losing control. I could no longer breathe in the manner I had been taught. During the breaks, I opened one eye and checked to see if I was still there.

I don't remember the midwife's name or face, but I do remember the things she said and did. During the childbirth preparation course that we had taken, the midwife in Beer Sheva had taught and encouraged me to pull myself upright while pushing to see the baby coming out. She told me these two attributes would allow me the special privilege and experience of witnessing my baby emerging from my body. For months I practiced and looked forward to this special moment.

What I remember most clearly about the midwife at the hospital was how she aggressively pushed me back down on the bed when I came forward for my big moment. She said that this action was not acceptable and that I could forget the fantasies I had fostered about viewing the birth. I lay back down on my back, stared at the ceiling, pushed my baby out and felt the shocking pain of the midwife's scissors cutting my body. I couldn't believe how much it hurt. And then I gave birth to my beautiful baby boy, my Udi. It was a truly amazing achievement, but it was tainted with feelings of disappointment, pain and violation.

The umbilical cord was wrapped around Udi's neck twice and was tied with two true knots. The midwife was horrified by thoughts of what might have happened and shouted to the other midwives to come to see the freak cord. I didn't quite understand what all the excitement was about. I wasn't a midwife then. I understand now. This birth could have ended tragically.

The suturing of the episiotomy was hellish and considerably more painful than the birth itself. No anesthetic was used. I tried to behave well but found it very difficult. Later I was cleaned up, placed on a gurney and wheeled off into a dark corridor. I was alone. Udi was in a plastic bassinet next to me, and I had no idea what to do.

I held him for a few minutes, and then he was taken away.

The only person I had contact with was an aide who put me on a bedpan, told me to pee and poured freezing cold water on my private parts. It was shocking. A few hours later when I got to the postpartum ward, Udi and I had our first true meeting, and he took the breast very eagerly. He was dark, with big black eyes and a pug nose. The mixture of our genes did an excellent job. I was in love.

Traumatic? Probably not. Warm and fuzzy? Absolutely not. Normal for the place and time? Probably. It saddens me to think how much potential joy was sucked out of the experience.

Up until Udi's birth I had never given much thought to the work that midwives do. I don't know if I even knew what a midwife was. Thoughts ran through my mind during the birth about the midwife and her job. I was awed just by the fact that she witnessed births daily and got paid to do so. It seemed like an incredibly cool way to make a living. On the other hand, I will never forget her brutality toward me. That shove to my chest remains with me to this day.

As a midwife, I have been told over and over throughout the years that this is not the way things are done here and that I can forget about my fantasies. Nevertheless, I continue to incessantly raise questions about the way things are done and to dream about how they could be better. That midwife pushed me down, but she certainly didn't knock me over.

My next pregnancy started when Udi was eleven months old. Avner and I were happy about the prospect of our two children being close in age, good friends and lifetime buddies. I was concerned about how Udi would accept his new sibling, and I suffered many sleepless nights over this issue. Other than that, my pregnancy was mostly carefree and eventless. We moved again and were living near the Sea of Galilee in a small settlement. I was outdoors with Udi most of the days; I felt like a truly natural woman, barefoot and pregnant, raising one baby while creating another.

Eitan was born at Poriya Hospital in Tiberias. I woke up one beautiful spring morning with very mild contractions. Again, I had completed 39 weeks and was exactly one week before my due date. As I went through my morning routine, I noticed that the contractions were regular but not painful. We decided to go to the hospital anyway, but on the way there I was filled with doubt. The timing and location of the contractions reminded me of my first labor, but there was no pain. The worst-case scenario was that they might send us home.

We arrived at the delivery room, and it was quiet and almost empty. Bilha, the midwife who greeted us, asked us why we came. I burst into laughter. Wasn't it obvious? Why would anyone come to the delivery room if not to have a baby? At the time I didn't know that there could be other reasons.

She checked me, and I was four centimeters dilated. I was stunned. I was still not experiencing any pain, and this incongruity left me confused and curious. This was nothing like my previous labor.

I asked a lot of questions. I mostly wanted to know if it was even possible to give birth to a baby without experiencing pain. The answer was noncommittal, that it is possible but not probable. We were told to go for a walk and to return when the contractions got stronger.

We went for a nice long walk. It was a warm spring day, and the grounds of the hospital were lovely. Everything was in bloom, and it was nice to be together, just the two of us. Udi was at home with his grandparents. After about two hours, I had to pee, and the contractions started to feel a bit stronger, so we went back. The midwife checked me again – seven centimeters! It was still hardly painful and barely believable. The midwife admitted me with a soapy warm water enema, a shave and a shower.

We were brought into a delivery room, and Bilha was there. She was the same midwife who had greeted us and had admitted me. I begged her not to cut me. The cut, the suturing and the recovery from the episiotomy from my first birth were some of the most difficult parts of my first birth experience. She promised me that if I listened to her instructions and cooperated with her, she would do everything in her power not to cut. This baby felt bigger than the first, and I hoped and prayed that I could avoid being cut. I liked her, and I trusted her. I believed that she would deliver the baby before her shift would end at 3 o'clock and that there would be no cutting.

She hooked me up to the monitor, and I was having impressive contractions every three minutes. She asked me if I agreed to have her break my waters. She explained that this could speed up the end of the labor and would ensure that she would deliver my baby. I agreed. I felt the hot water rushing out of my body, and I understood that there was no going back. The contractions became very powerful very quickly.

Within half an hour I was fully dilated, and ten minutes later I was pushing. I listened to her every word knowing that the integrity of my perineum depended on my obedience. Eitan was born as if he had been pushed down a well-greased slide. He weighed 3.990 kg; there were no cuts, no scratches, no tears, not even a drop of blood. Ten minutes later

I pushed the placenta out, and he took the breast immediately into his mouth and started sucking. This was a very different experience from my first birth. I was exhilarated. This was easy; this was actually fun! This was the natural birth that I had fantasized about. Bilha was my friend, my cohort, my heroine!

It was a bit of a roller coaster ride at the end, but it was over. Clearly, there were no traumas in this birth experience. It was almost too good to be true. A few hours later, I declared to my family that I felt so good that I was ready to go out dancing at a discotheque; it was the 80s.

Again, just like after Udi's birth, the image of the midwife permeated my thoughts whenever I recalled my birth experience. Those midwives were relaxed and confident; they sent me to the garden to walk; I was barely on the monitor; they took control of the situation, and they helped me to have my baby the way I wanted to. I don't even remember seeing a doctor during Eitan's birth. My memory of the midwife is the memory of a strong and independent woman who knew what she was doing and who knew secrets about the way babies are born. I wanted to be that woman. I wanted to learn the secrets that she knew.

Yael was born two years and two months later at HaEmek Hospital in Afula. Udi was almost four years old, and Eitan was two years and two months old. Again, 39 weeks, again exactly one week before my due date. Labor started in the morning, and we drove to the hospital. Both Avner and I were expecting an easy birth just like the last one.

I was admitted with regular contractions with a dilation of four centimeters. As with my previous birth, I was sent for a walk, but it was too hot to go outside. During the walk through the corridors, the labor didn't progress. I was called back into the delivery room and was notified that a decision had been made to augment my labor with Pitocin because they needed the bed. I had no idea what this meant, but I agreed. I was losing my patience with being pregnant and wanted to have my baby.

I had done a pretty good job in the past and had no reason to believe that this experience would be any different from the others.

I soon discovered that this was far from the truth. After the needle of the IV was stuck in my arm, I was hooked up to the monitor and asked to lie on my side. The Pitocin began to drip into my vein, and the contractions picked up in their frequency and intensity. I can't remember how long it took until I was having contractions every two minutes. As soon as one contraction ended, the next one began. Again, I felt like a knife had been thrust into my back, but this time it was serrated.

Avner was not aware of the pain I was feeling. He was acting as if I was in Poriya at Eitan's almost painless birth. He was drinking coffee and schmoozing with the staff. The midwife came into the room every once in a while to check the monitor and offer me painkilling drugs. The idea of drugs seemed absurd to me; after two natural births, why would I want to take drugs? I refused. And she offered again, and I refused again. And on and on. I was in a kind of Hell. There was no exit, no solution and no end to the suffering. I remember begging Avner to take me home. I was afraid that this would never end. There was no laughter in this birth, no joy, no nature, no cooperation. I just wanted it to be over.

At some point, the midwife entered the room with a syringe and injected its contents into the IV fluids going into my vein. She didn't tell me what it was, and I didn't ask. This is the last thing I clearly remember from Yael's birth. I don't remember pushing; I don't remember when she came out. I do remember that she was beautiful and looked like a little Japanese doll. I remember the feeling of relief. I remember asking myself, "What the f*** was that?" I remember being angry for being made to feel this way.

The next day I went back to the delivery room and gave the midwife a box of chocolates. For the life of me, to this day, I don't know why. Maybe because she didn't cut me or push me. Maybe because she cared enough to offer me drugs. Maybe because she was just doing her job, and I appreciated that. Maybe I just didn't want the chocolates.

This experience is clearly one of the sources of my sensitivity to the emotional aspects of the birth experience. Women giving birth should not feel anger, fear, weakness, vulnerability or disconnection. They should be filled with love, expectation, capability, connection and faith.

Was this birth experience traumatic? A bit. Now that I understand more about trauma, I see that some of the defining elements were present: helplessness, overwhelming emotion, fear, loss of control and loneliness. Like most women, I got over it. I had three small kids to raise; it helped that I had a supportive family and lived in a close community. Five days after Yael's birth, we all went to my brother-in-law's wedding. As I said earlier, I was young, strong and healthy.

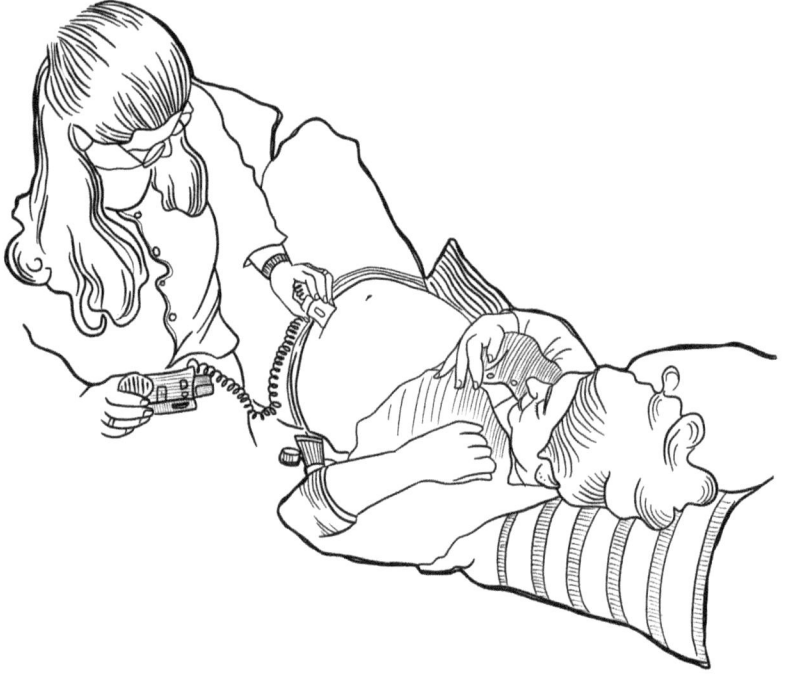

Becoming Mindwife

.

My continuing search for the connection between birth and trauma beckons me to explore the experience of my birth when I was born in 1955. My knowledge is limited because my mother didn't recall much despite my persistent attempts to prod her memory. Her lack of recall may indicate that drugs had been administered. A combination of drugs nicknamed "Twilight Sleep" was very much in style at the time.

What she did tell me was that her pregnancy with me was unplanned and unwanted. I was the fifth child, and she already had one or two too many children. A fifth was more than she could or wanted to manage.

She made several attempts to abort the pregnancy but to no avail. She hid the pregnancy from her relatives, friends and neighbors until the seventh month hoping it would somehow go away, but it didn't. I survived the pregnancy and had an unmemorable birth. I believe that somewhere, embedded deeply in my body are two terrifying sensations: the threat of annihilation and the feeling of not being wanted, a pretty traumatic way to begin life.

I continued to put together pieces of the puzzle and how this has shaped who I became as a daughter, a sister, a woman, a friend, a mother, a partner, a midwife and a trauma therapist. The narrative of my life story is a quest to justify my existence and to prove to my mother and the world, but mostly to myself, that I am a worthwhile, useful and significant human being. This pursuit for significance set me on a course that led me to leave America, move to Israel, marry an Israeli man, give birth to three babies in four years and become a midwife, a teacher and a trauma therapist.

When my children were five, seven and nine years old I enrolled in nursing school intending to subsequently study midwifery and become a midwife. I became certified as a nurse after studying for three and a half years, worked with premature and sick newborns in the Neonatal Intensive Care Unit for a year and a half and then completed an advanced nursing degree in Midwifery. The entire process took six years.

I worked in the labor and delivery unit for nine years where I developed professionally and became a confident and knowledgeable midwife. I learned something new from every woman I cared for, and I loved every minute of it. I was often quoted as saying, "I love it so much that I would happily do it without even being paid."

I loved the women, the dynamics of the couples and the different languages and cultures. I loved being part of a team, working shoulder to shoulder with other midwives, women helping women, doing women's work. I loved the challenges, the drama, the intimacy and the babies. I even loved being with women in the unfortunate circumstances of intrapartum death, premature deliveries and emergency C-sections. I felt needed; I felt significant. My life was filled with meaning. I knew that I was making a difference in the lives of these women. I felt that my presence was preventing the formation of traumatic birth experiences.

My clinical instructor, Nitza, taught me everything she knew and loved about midwifery. She exemplified the fusion of theoretical knowledge and emotional intelligence that the ideal midwife should possess, and she did everything in her power to pass that on to me. She always saw the woman as being the locus of control, and this was an infinitely valuable lesson that she imparted to me. She was a closet feminist and my mentor. She taught me to listen deeply to the women because they knew better than anyone else what they needed. We are still good friends.

With time I too became a clinical instructor, and when Nitza left her post, I replaced her as assistant to the head midwife and initiated many projects and innovations. After six years, I began teaching midwifery in the same school for advanced nursing studies where I had studied and thus gained a new perspective by stepping outside of the Labor and Delivery Unit (L&D).

I began to see the health system from a broader viewpoint; I traveled abroad to attend conferences and met midwifery educators from other countries. I helped to create study programs and wrote questions for national certification exams. In the process, I met and got to know many midwives from other delivery rooms in the country. Midwifery wasn't just a job for me; it was becoming a career.

I needed a Master's degree to move forward in any way, and I couldn't continue teaching without going back to school. I searched high and low until I found the right program and eventually registered at the Israeli extension of Lesley College for a Master's program in Women's Studies. There I discovered that I was a feminist which for me meant that I was a woman working with women, doing women's work, for the benefit of women and empowering women in any way I could.

During my second year of study at Lesley College, I wrote a thesis on the topic of trauma and birth, specifically about the birth experiences of women who had been the victims of terrorist bombings. I interviewed women who had had the misfortune of having been present at bombing incidents and subsequently gave birth, some several months later, some after many years. I explored, together with them, the connections between the trauma of the incident and their experiences of pregnancy, birth and mothering.

I learned a lot more about trauma than I had expected to and was strongly pulled into its vortex for over a year. I met with eight brave women who, above all, taught me that life goes on even after horrendous things happen, that children are a force of nature, that we are capable of a lot more healing than we can ever imagine and that birth is truly a focal event in women's lives.

An Excerpt from my Thesis Journal

Today I met with Shulamit Saban. She is 47 years old, married and the mother of four children, two sons and two daughters, ages 26, 20, 17 and 11. She has lived all her life in Sfat, a city in northern Israel. She is a special education teacher by profession, and she works as the supervisor and coordinator of all special education programs and teachers in the district surrounding Sfat.

Thirty years ago in 1974, when Shulamit was 16 years old, she was taken hostage by terrorists, together with 105 classmates and ten teachers during a school outing in an incident that has come to be known as "The Ma'alot Massacre." Twenty-one students and three teachers were killed, and 68 others were injured by automatic rifle fire and hand grenade explosions. Israeli soldiers attempted to free the hostages from the kidnappers who had held them hostage for over 12 hours. During the crossfire between the soldiers and the terrorists, Shulamit saved her own life by jumping out of a second-story window. She woke up two days later with a severely fractured arm and internal injuries in her lungs and intestines.

Shulamit was hospitalized for over two months and underwent a series of operations and years of physical therapy and rehabilitation. She never regained the full use of her right arm.

Three years after the incident at age 19, Shulamit married the man who helped nurse her back to health, a young soldier who never left her side throughout the pain, trauma, loneliness and fears that persisted long after the physical scars healed. Shulamit had serious doubts that she would ever be able to have children, a thought that went through her head even as she contemplated jumping from the window.

A few months after the wedding, she was overjoyed to discover that she was pregnant. Pregnancy, she felt, was her means of defeating the terrorists. She hoped that by becoming a mother she would find a way to create a normal life like other normal Israeli women. Continuing to suffer pain and disability in her injured right arm, Shulamit was particularly fearful that her pregnancy would not go to full term because of the multiple adhesions in her abdomen.

The pregnancy did go to full term. During two days in labor Shulamit relived the terrorist incident over and over as she gave birth to her son. When the time came to push her baby out, the midwives encouraged her by calling, "Push, push, push!" All she could hear was, "Jump, jump, jump!" As her baby was born, she felt herself flying through the air between the window and the ground. The two experiences had blended into one. If I had any doubts about whether or not there is a connection between birth and trauma, Shulamit taught me that there most definitely is.

As a new mother, she was paralyzed by insecurities, memories of the trauma and fear. She sought help and entered therapy that continued for six years until she felt secure enough to have another child. In 1990 Shulamit published her diary entitled **To Live Again**. *Today, thirty years after the incident, she is still haunted by her memories.*

Shulamit Saban was my first interviewee; this was my pilot study. I remember standing by my car after completing the interview, not knowing what to do with myself, who to call, or how to put into words what I had just heard. I had been a witness to a first-hand account of the blending that can take place between the memory of a traumatic event and a birth experience. My suspicions were justified; my intuitions had been accurate. I received the push I needed to go forward and find more women, hear more stories, learn more about this and tell the world.

I went on to find seven additional women who bravely opened up their homes and their hearts. It was not an easy time for me. Their stories and the images they conjured up haunted my thoughts by day and my dreams at night. These women were with me for a year, and my interactions with them helped me to gain a new perspective on my own life and my own traumas.

In writing my thesis I acquired a tremendous amount of theoretical knowledge about trauma, post-trauma, PTSD, posttraumatic growth and various healing modalities. This new knowledge, together with the stories of my interviewees, took up most of the available space in my mind. I had trauma on my mind most of the time.

After I submitted my Master's thesis, I felt a huge sense of relief, and my mind cleared. I went back to the delivery room and noticed that it had begun to feel like a cage. I felt stifled, unable to express myself, incapable of using my knowledge and my skills. My level of frustration rose, and there were days when I wanted to scream. There was so much work and so little time to be with the women who needed me.

I found myself saying over and over again, "I'll be right back." Sometimes I was too busy to come back, or I would come back a whole lot later than I had intended to. Then I would apologize for disappearing for so long, and the women would seem to be okay with it because they didn't expect more from the medical system. Was this the best way to bring new babies into the world? Expecting little and getting even less? How much lower would we go? What did the women expect from the staff? Very little and then they would settle for even less.

I started asking myself if I wanted to be a part of a system that dictates its priorities according to statistics, the average woman and the average birth. Who is the average woman anyway? What is her name? Where does she live? How does she feel about giving birth? Does she know the power and wisdom of her own body? Is she so scared of anything that is uncomfortable that she needs the average epidural to numb her average senses and wait for her average womb to try hard to get her average baby out of her average pelvis and meet this average world? Is this it? Could we do better? Could I do better?

Journal Entry: Searching for Connections

I am still struggling with my connection between trauma and birth. I have been reading over my thesis, going back through the materials and doing a lot of thinking and writing about these topics. I have lectured at Midwifery conferences about the birth experiences of terrorist bombing survivors. The audiences were moved by the stories. The reactions of the midwives indicated to me that this was a topic that needed to be further explored. They even waited in line during the coffee break to talk with me about their experiences. They had been there; they had delivered the babies of posttraumatic women and understood what I was talking about.

I am intensely reading Penny Simkin's book **When Survivors Give Birth** *on the birth experiences of childhood sexual abuse survivors. It is as if she has read my thesis. Our findings are astoundingly similar even though the traumas are different. I am beginning to understand that the manifestations of trauma are universal and expressed in the pathophysiology of the body. The content of the trauma seems to matter less than how the body reacts to it. While doing research for my thesis, I encountered this approach in Peter Levine's book* **Waking the Tiger**, *and it sparked my interest then and even more so now.*

I have also been examining my own curiosity about this topic, and I keep digging and digging inside myself, each time finding another small piece of the puzzle that somehow connects me with the traumas of women. It continues to baffle me, and I remain curious and continue to explore.

I asked myself many times if, as a child, I experienced anything that might qualify as abuse. What comes to mind over and over is my relationship with my older brothers. When we were young there was a lot of teasing, fighting, tickle torture, wrestling and in general, situations in which I felt weak and helpless. There is a fine line between innocent rough play between siblings and cruelty, and sometimes it felt like perhaps that line had been crossed. I adored my brothers; they were demigods for me. I spent much more time with them than with anyone else, including my parents.

My love, my age and my devotion to them made me vulnerable to their overzealous roughhousing. Today I understand that I was mistreated, maybe even abused. Today I understand that the line had been crossed, even though it was most probably unintentional. Today I understand that I saw myself as a victim, and they were at the same time, both my saviors and my abusers.

I was younger than they were, weaker than they were. They were two, and I was one. They were boys, and I was a girl. I was knocked down every time I tried to rise up, and despite the degradation, I continued to seek their approval, their permission, their attention and their love. I grew up, and I was shaped by these yearnings. Parts of me aimed to please; I learned to fear those who have authority and power over me. I learned to make do in challenging situations, rarely pursuing confrontation and never rocking the boat.

I never spoke about any of this with anyone then and never complained to my parents. This was a secret I kept because I was afraid that I would pay the price if I told. To a very small but certain extent, I tasted what abuse feels like, along with the fear, the loneliness, the distrust and the helplessness that go along with it.

I started working with women privately, listening to their stories and preparing them for their births in the best way I could. Most of these women were posttraumatic. Some of their traumas were the result of adverse childhood events: sometimes from a car accident or being thrown off a horse. Sometimes the trauma was the result of growing up with Holocaust survivors. But most often the trauma was the result of a previous birth: an emergency C-section, vacuum delivery, premature birth or stillbirth.

The potential for the manifestation of traumatic events in the delivery room is huge. No one who is present is immune, not even the woman who washes the floor. Sometimes, as the midwife, I participated in difficult births and suffered afterward from sleepless nights, flashbacks, avoidant behavior and hypervigilance. The more I learned about trauma the more I realized how difficult it is to work in the delivery room.

I observed behaviors in myself and in my colleagues that can only be explained as being generated by posttraumatic reactions to difficult events.

I began studying Somatic Experiencing (SE), a mind-body healing modality based on a model created by Peter Levine. One of the basic premises of SE is that trauma manifests itself in the body as energy that becomes stuck, usually as the result of a freeze reaction to a surprising and life-threatening event. Another premise is that the body naturally wants to heal itself, and the healing process can be enabled by bringing attention to the trapped energy and allowing the body to organically discharge it. As I continued my studies and learned more about trauma, I also learned more about birth, as both a potentially healing and potentially traumatizing event.

Journal Entry: What I Have Learned about Birth by Studying about Trauma

Birth has a rhythm of its own. Each woman experiences it differently. Each woman sings her own birth song and dances her own birth dance. Afterward, she often finds it difficult to put into words what the experience felt like, what emotions were stirred, where the black holes that she fell into, the brick walls she faced and the enlightened moments of elation and grace that flowed through and around her. Birth is an experience of the body, and the body knows how to give birth. The same is true of trauma and healing.

Each of us experiences trauma differently in a very personal and individual manner with a rhythm and a tempo of our own. The fear and anxiety, together with the joy and pleasure that the body experiences, are all felt inherently in the muscles, joints and viscera. The body knows how to release trapped traumatic energy, but the mind doesn't always allow it to do so or even know how to describe it.

Both birth and trauma are experiences of the body. Both involve intimate communication with the body, basic instinctual behavior controlled by the most primitive parts of the brain. Two basic needs, to survive and to reproduce, express themselves intuitively through the body. The expression of these basic needs through the wisdom of the body frees us from the tethers of the mind. Experiencing the powerful wisdom of the body can be exhilarating.

The approach to dealing with the challenges of birth must be personal. Each woman experiences birth from her own special perspective of the world. Her birth will be an honest and direct reflection of who she is. There is no "package deal" for birth preparation. Each woman needs a personal fitting for her birth, like a bride and her customized wedding dress. The art of helping a woman prepare for childbirth involves helping her to identify her resources: her inner strengths, her support systems, her way of being talked to, her way of being touched.

Trauma healing is deep work, as is preparing for childbirth, giving birth and becoming a mother. Giving birth is like becoming the epicenter of an earthquake. The baby, an entire human being who has taken up residence inside the womb, has to negotiate the bones of her mother's pelvis in order to make the passage. It is an earth-shaking event. It rocks the mother to her core. When we heal our trauma, we give birth to ourselves. We push through the bones of our histories, shaking our earth and searching for new air to breathe.

Why has birth become such a traumatizing event? In this age of technological, medicalized hospital birth, women often find themselves shocked and surprised by the nature of their birth experiences. For many of them, it is the first time they step foot in a hospital. Their naive expectation is for a pink and fuzzy experience, and the reality turns out to be painted a very different color.

Many women give birth on their backs immobilized by doctors, nurses and/or midwives standing over them, shouting at them to push, holding their legs open while doing so. If their bodies are numbed by epidurals, they are hindered in succeeding to do what they are told because of the lack of feedback they are getting from their bodies. Women are often told that their babies are in distress and that emergency procedures must be performed in order to save their lives. In comes the terror. Women in labor are often abused verbally, treated like children and ignored; their needs are disregarded, and their feelings are discounted. In comes the rage.

They can neither fight nor flee, so their bodies freeze. They are forced to keep going and don't have the opportunity to collapse and recover from the freeze. Women's needs and requests are ignored. It often seems like birth workers are willing to do everything and anything in their power to get the baby out. The natural birth process is often sabotaged. Add on vacuum deliveries, episiotomies, emergency C-sections, helpless and enraged partners and babies in NICU. The list is long.

So how can birth be healing? Like effective trauma healing, a physiological birth takes place gradually. The contractions build when the mother is ready. As the contractions get stronger, her capacity to contain the pain increases. The uterus contracts and expands intermittently in waves. This rhythm creates an opportunity to rest and integrate each contraction before the next one arrives. The deeper the relaxation, the more effective the contractions. If the birthing woman is surrounded by support, patience and love, a safe atmosphere is created and there is space for healing.

In a good birth, the woman is open and willing to accept whatever may come up for her during the process. There is no fear of the pain. Instead, there is curiosity and acceptance. Deep listening to the body guides the process. As the labor progresses, the listening gets deeper, and the woman enters a dream-like state. Dual awareness is maintained; the woman is tuned into her inner self and at the same time knows exactly what she needs from those surrounding her. Time loses its meaning. Movement, vocalization and communication become reptilian. Danger is sensed intuitively and successfully avoided. There is trust and belief in the process. There is potential and possibility for transformation.

Pushing the baby out requires a concerted physical effort, deep concentration and focus. Along with contractions of the uterus and the pushing efforts of the mother, there is often sweating, trembling, tears, shouting and grunting. Everything that was inside goes out. There is an enormous feeling of satisfaction, relief and discharge when the baby is born. The sensations in the afterglow of birth include wellbeing, calm, heat and energy flow.

I tried to incorporate these understandings into my work. My attempts at being a better-than-average trauma-aware midwife were often problematic. When I tried to do my best, when I tried to be creative within the walls of the delivery room, I met a lot of opposition. I had more success when the doctors were sleeping, when they were at staff meetings or when they were busy taking care of someone who actually needed their expertise, such as a sick woman who needed medical attention.

Then I could be inventive. I could try out new things that I had learned. I could do radical things like letting the woman get out of bed and sit on a chair or a ball or eat or take a nice long shower or push standing up or on hands-and-knees or go to the toilet with a large dilation. These were revolutionary actions and needed to be done underground, not in the light of day, not under the direct gaze of the authoritative, cynical, misogynistic, sarcastic or distrustful.

Push came to shove after a very memorable night shift. One of the women in my care had been in bed all day on a fetal monitor with an intravenous Pitocin drip. She was miserable. Her back ached, and all she wanted was to stand up, stretch her body, eat something and go to the bathroom to pee. She felt horrible just from lying down all day. I stopped the Pitocin, released her from the monitor and sent her to the shower and the toilet. She ate something and felt like a human being again. She sat on a birthing ball and slowly allowed some movement to enter her hips. A smile spread over her face, her color returned to her cheeks and her mood improved. I reconnected her to the Pitocin drip and the fetal monitor. There was a clear and reassuring reading of normal fetal heart rate and regular contractions on the strip.

One of the doctors was doing rounds, and when he came into the room, he immediately expressed his disapproval of her use of the birth ball and asked me to return the woman to the bed. This seemed to be such a shame; she was upright, on the monitor, on the drip. What was the problem? An argument ensued and with it, elevated levels of loud disagreement between us. He wanted her in bed. I tried to understand the difference between sitting in the bed and sitting on a ball or on a chair. As far as he was concerned, there was a world of difference. He ordered me to get her back into bed and emphasized that, on principle, it was actually just because he had said so. It was the doctor's orders. She begged me to let go of the argument. She would do as he said. She didn't want me to get into trouble on her account.

I was disappointed with her obedience and that she didn't fight at all for her right to be upright and out of bed. I was frustrated and could feel my body becoming enraged in reaction to the doctor's inflexible attitude. I knew that birth progresses better when women are upright and mobile, and I understood that he desperately needed to feel in control, but I was unable to communicate all of this at the time. I felt the words stuck in my throat, and they were never expressed. I am clearly not at my best in situations that involve confrontation and authority.

When that shift ended, I knew that my days in the delivery room were numbered. I couldn't do this anymore. My health was on the line. It was making me sick. I could no longer watch birthing women hand over their power and the control of their bodies to perfect strangers. I was no longer willing to stand by and watch women abused and disempowered. If I couldn't be part of the solution, then I was a part of the problem, and that was unacceptable to me. I decided to leave the hospital and become a home birth midwife. Out of the hospital I would be able to be truer to myself.

My convictions and confidence were both in direct confrontation with my fears. This inner confrontation would continue to accompany me for many years. This was a leap of faith for me: faith in women's bodies, faith in the birthing process, faith in nature and faith in my ability to know safety from danger, normal from pathology. I would miss the team of midwives with whom I had worked for years, but I would never miss the politics, the power struggles, the violence, the lies or the threats. I would be on my own, and I would do things my way.

As part of creating a home birth business, I created a new email account. An idea for my new address jumped into my head: mindwife@gmail.com. It expressed exactly what I was feeling, that my Self and my profession had finally become one.

Eventually, I began to feel like a bird that had been released from its cage. It took time before I could feel the expanse of my wings, spread them open and really learn to fly, but eventually, I did. One of the places my wings took me to was to Africa. I spent six weeks in Tanzania, Ethiopia and South Africa. I lived with midwives there, taught them what I knew and learned about their lives. I learned about the obstacles they face, trying to do their work without minimal resources like clean, running water, passable roads and basic medical supplies.

I learned about their lives as women, often abandoned by their men, raising children alone, working and fending for themselves. I learned about the real, day-to-day threats of diseases like malaria, AIDS and yellow fever, along with the newer medical realities of hypertension, diabetes and heart disease. Africa left a lasting impression on me. When I got home, I marveled at the fact that I could drink the water in my shower, that not only was it clean, but it was also hot and running. Africa helped me to appreciate what I have, what we all have, including access to doctors and hospitals.

For ten of the fifteen years during which I was doing home births, I also had a very special arrangement with the Scottish Hospital in Nazareth. Because it was a private facility, I was able to transfer my home birth clients who required a higher level of care and also continue to function as their midwife. In addition, I brought in private clients and cared for them in the delivery room.

This enabled me to provide continuous care to clients who were categorized as high risk and did not meet the criteria for a home birth. I could now do prenatal, intrapartum and postpartum care with women after Cesareans and women with gestational diabetes, prolonged rupture of membranes, oligo – and polyhydramnios, big babies, small babies, premature babies, clotting abnormalities, etc. It was a terrific arrangement while it lasted. And I loved working with the midwives and doctors from a culture that was very different from mine. I was still in Israel, but working in Nazareth was like visiting a friendly and familiar foreign country half an hour from my home.

The hospital administration changed and with it, the director of the delivery room. Unfortunately, they did not recognize the advantages of this service, and it was eliminated.

For fifteen years I was on call for out-of-hospital births and/or private in-hospital births in Nazareth, often four or five at once. I became an active member of Imahi, the Israeli organization of homebirth midwives. I continued to teach young, aspiring midwives, imparting to them some of the clinical knowledge that I acquired throughout the years. I became a certified Body-Mind Psychotherapist and opened a clinic specializing in work with women who were suffering from post-trauma by helping them prepare for healing and empowering births. Some of these women birthed with me; some did not.

After 15 years of working outside the hospital and accompanying women to 444 births, I decided that it was time to stop. This was a much more difficult decision for me to make than leaving the hospital; it felt like I was removing an organ from my body. I had become Mindwife; there was no longer a separation between the woman and the profession. I was a midwife 24 hours a day, seven days a week.

I felt the need to get back to being just me by inviting the midwife to retire. The therapist is still flourishing, as is the teacher, the grandmother, the mother and the wife. And the writer is finding her voice.

Today, I am doing one-on-one supervision with birth professionals, lecturing and facilitating group seminars and workshops in an attempt to spread my knowledge about trauma, post-trauma and complex PTSD to midwives, nurses, doctors, doulas and anyone else who wants to learn.

Even though the midwife has retired, she is alive and kicking deep inside of me. I am proud to continue to call myself a home birth midwife. It will always be a part of who I am.

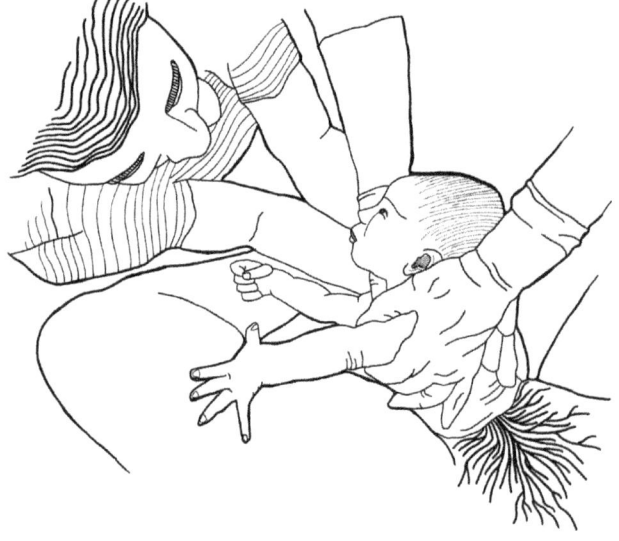

Learning to Listen to Women in the Delivery Room

When I was a midwifery student, I was afforded the luxury of taking care of one woman at a time. Every once in a while, toward the end of my training, I would take on the challenge of caring for two women simultaneously.

Only Six Centimeters

One of those days came when I felt confident and ready to care for two women. In one room there was a woman in her first pregnancy, being induced with Pitocin because her pregnancy had gone beyond her due date. I checked in on her intermittently to make sure that she was comfortable, that the drip was working properly, that the fetal monitor was reassuring and that her contractions were slowly increasing in their frequency and amplitude.

In the adjacent room was an older religious woman who was laboring with her seventh baby. We chatted about her previous births, and she told me that I should know that she gives birth when she is six centimeters dilated. As a midwifery student, I felt obligated to explain to her that no one gives birth with a dilation less than ten centimeters, that this is the diameter of the baby's head and that it can't pass through the cervix with an opening smaller than that. She insisted that with each baby, she had given birth with six centimeters and that this is a fact.

As time went by, I went back and forth between the two rooms. In one room a young couple with no birth experience was anxiously waiting for the birth to begin. In the other room a woman with a lot of birth experience was alone in the dark, coping with the pain and waiting for it to end.

At one point, the contractions got a little stronger, and the experienced birther asked me to examine her; she was six centimeters dilated. I made a mental note that she was entering active labor and decided that I should check on her neighbor in case things picked up quickly.

While I was in the adjacent room, I heard an audible pop and dashed back in. What was before me? Her bed was drenched in a sea of amniotic fluid, flowing off the bedsheets and onto the floor, and in the middle of the puddle was a wet, cold, screaming baby.

I was, needless to say, speechless. The speed of the incident was alarming. I put on a pair of gloves, separated the umbilical cord, handed her the baby and cleaned up the mess, feeling both stupid and humiliated. All the time, she kept chuckling and telling me over and over, "I told you I give birth at six centimeters. You should have listened to me." **That was the first and last time I argued with a woman in labor**. I am happy that I learned this very important lesson before I received my license to practice midwifery.

Lesson learned:
1. I should have listened.
2. I have a lot to learn.
3. There is no point arguing with a laboring woman.
4. Women know themselves and their bodies. I need to stop thinking that I know about labor from what I learned in school and start learning everything I can from the women themselves.
5. There is no such thing as labor "by the book."

More Luck than Brains

When I first started working in the hospital, I was under the direct supervision of an experienced midwife for two months until I was trusted to work alone. Then I was encouraged to continue to ask for help or supervision as complicated situations arose. My first night shift on my own was a busy one. Altogether, we were three midwives covering triage, six delivery rooms and two pre-labor beds.

One of the women I was caring for was a very tall woman carrying a baby with an estimated weight of four kilograms. The birthing unit was filled to capacity, and women seemed to be having babies in every room. Even the doctors were doing normal deliveries, which was a rare situation. I went from room to room, trying to find someone to be with me (because of the high weight estimation), but no one was free. I resigned myself to the fact that I would be doing this birth on my own. I could feel my pulse racing, and I tried to calm myself, as I could feel the adrenaline rushing through my body.

I prepared to receive the baby double-checking everything to make sure I hadn't forgotten any equipment. I understood that no one would even be free to respond to a cry for help if I needed it.

Then the baby started coming and kept coming and coming. The head was massive, but it slipped gracefully out and into my hands. The shoulders were chubby, but they also came out without any problem. Then I held him in my hands and found myself looking down at the biggest newborn baby I had ever seen. He was huge. I handed him to his mother who welcomed her into her arms while trying to manage her own shocked reaction to his size. He looked like a two-month-old.

When I placed him on the scale. He weighed 4.700 kg. (10 lbs. 6 oz.). My body started to tremble as catastrophic thoughts raced through my mind and fear clenched my chest over what could have happened to the baby (shoulder dystocia) or the mother (a severe perineal tear or post-partum hemorrhage), what might happen to me when this information gets out (being reprimanded) and why was I alone with all this? I kept looking at the baby and mother in an attempt to convince my fears that everything was okay and that no catastrophes had actually happened. She hadn't even torn. Slowly my body calmed down.

I wanted to tell everyone and simultaneously wanted no one to know. There was something shameful about being a part of something so out of the ordinary. When I finally joined the veteran midwives at the nursing station who were all documenting births, I blurted out the baby's birth weight. Their eyes popped out of their sockets. And, the most senior among them said something to me that I will never forget, "You have more luck than brains."

I was insulted then, but now I think that maybe she was right. I hoped then, and still hope now, that I have both luck and brains.

Lessons Learned:
1. She was right – I did have more luck than brains.
2. Luck and brains create a good equation for a successful midwifery career.
3. Beginner's luck helps.
4. That baby, that mother and I managed to slip under the radar of the fear that often comes with too much knowledge.

Journal Entry: Honoring Intuition

I was working an evening shift in the delivery room. There was a phone call from a nurse on the obstetric ward. She wanted to speak to a doctor. There were no doctors in the immediate vicinity; the midwife who answered the phone told her to try the physician's beeper and hung up the phone. The same nurse called again five minutes later and asked to speak to a doctor. I took the receiver and asked her what the problem was. She was concerned about a woman in her 26th week of pregnancy who was complaining of severe abdominal pain. Something in her voice caused me to take action.

I hung up the phone, and without saying a word to anyone, quickly took a pair of gloves, a delivery set and a cord clamp and went to the obstetric ward. Behind my back, I could hear comments and questions about what I was doing, where I was going and why I was taking all this equipment with me.

It was visiting hours in the obstetric ward, and through the crowds of families and friends, I was ushered to the bed of the aforementioned woman by the nurse who had phoned. The woman was writhing in pain, biting her lips and on the verge of tears. She didn't say much but had terror in her eyes. I asked her to remove her underpants so I could examine her. As she parted her legs, I saw through the slightly opened outer lips of her vagina what appeared to be the head of her baby.

Within seconds, the baby was on its way out and into my gloved hand. It weighed about 700 grams, gave a weak cry and then was quiet. I quickly separated the umbilical cord and wrapped the baby in several layers of sheeting; I immediately started a heart massage with one finger on its tiny fragile chest. I headed for the Neonatal Intensive Care Unit. I could hear my own heart pounding.

The baby survived after several months in the NICU. The mother had already lost two babies in premature labor. This one survived.

I cannot explain rationally why I went off to the obstetric ward in the manner in which I did. Something inside me spoke to me and led me through the actions I took.

Lessons learned:
1. Even though I was surprised when the baby slipped into my hands, somehow, I knew this was going to happen.
2. Intuition is a precious tool in this profession and needs to be respected.
3. Sometimes it is difficult to understand exactly what it is that my intuition is trying to tell me. I do know that every time I paid attention and listened, exercised caution or acted, the outcome was always better. I never regretted listening to my intuition, though I have regretted ignoring it.

Too Busy to Birth

During the early part of an evening shift, a woman walked into the triage of the L&D. She had a compact pregnant belly and was smartly dressed in a skirt suit and high heels. She looked very businesslike and not at all in labor. She proclaimed as she walked in the door, "I came in because they told me to. I was in the middle of a meeting, and all the women there told me that I should go to the hospital because I look like I'm in labor. I don't know what they are talking about."

We went through the usual process: urine test for protein, blood pressure, fetal monitor, vaginal exam, ultrasound. She did not have any documentation of her pregnancy with her; she had come straight from work. She assured me that everything was OK. On the monitor, there were contractions every three minutes, which she didn't feel at all. When I checked her cervix, I was shocked. It was six centimeters dilated, she was fully effaced and the head was pushing down on it forcefully.

I explained to her that she was in active labor and that she would be giving birth soon. At first, she argued with me that this couldn't possibly be and that she had to get back to work. Then, as the reality of the situation started to filter in, she realized that she had to call her husband who was also at work so that he could join her. She still sounded doubtful in their phone conversation, but he was on his way.

She got out of her high heels, changed into a hospital gown and slowly started to feel the contractions. As we filled in the forms for her admission, the contractions became more and more present, more and more uncomfortable for her. She transformed into a woman in labor right before my eyes.

By the time we finished the admission process and she got settled in one of the delivery rooms, she was groaning and whimpering and asking for an epidural because she was experiencing intense physical pain. Not more than a half-hour had gone by since her arrival. By the time her husband joined us, she had an intravenous line in her arm, she was hooked up to the fetal monitor and she was begging for the anesthesiologist to come to administer an epidural. An hour had not yet passed since the moment she had stepped foot in triage. She got her epidural and gave birth within an hour.

After the baby was in her arms, we all started processing what had happened. She realized that if she had waited longer at work, she might have had the baby there or on the way in an ambulance, and her husband might have missed out.

My thoughts went in a completely different direction. I was in awe of what I had just witnessed: the power of the mind over the body.

Lessons learned:

1. The thing we call attention or intention has a very powerful influence on the body.
2. The moment she realized that she was in labor the contractions started to become painful. As she brought her attention to the pain, it increased. Up until then, her attention had been elsewhere and she had experienced no pain whatsoever.
3. Where we focus our attention determines how we experience ourselves in the present time.
4. Pain is a subjective experience that is influenced by many factors, both conscious and unconscious.
5. It is impossible to imagine how another person experiences pain. It is such a personal and unique experience.

Natural Twins

I remember a Russian woman in her first pregnancy with twins. From week 35 she was told to come in once a week for a check-up. Every week the findings were the same; her babies were fine and she was healthy. Each time, she was given "permission" to let the pregnancy continue for another week, and each week, she told the doctors and midwives that she wasn't asking for permission. She wanted a natural birth; she was not interested in any interventions or manipulations and she knew that her babies were just fine. She continued to come, and the ritual repeated itself each week.

And then she disappeared. Her last visit had been at week 39. We all assumed that she had switched hospitals. No one gave her too much thought until she showed up with contractions.

She was then in week 41, her babies were both positioned with their heads down, with weight estimations over three kilograms and she was in active labor. When I saw her, I smiled to myself. Her determination and belief in herself caused me to feel pride in birthing women everywhere. She had been adamant about birthing naturally when her babies were ripe and ready, and here she was.

She seemed to be in great physical, emotional and mental shape, almost superhuman. And I had the fortune to take care of her. Her babies were fine. Both of their pulses remained normal throughout the labor, and she was amazing. She was quiet, almost stoic, patient and attentive to herself. She managed to move as much as she possibly could. Her husband was loving and supportive; they spoke Russian throughout the labor. It was like a movie without subtitles. I couldn't understand a word they spoke, but I was hypnotized.

Twin births are usually very popular and crowded affairs. The attendees usually include: at least two midwives , at least two OBs, two pediatricians and various additional onlookers, such as nursing students, midwifery students and medical students.

The mother of these twins expressed over and over again that she wanted as few people in the room as possible. I apologized and explained that the protocol is in place to ensure maximum safety and optimal care. And then the birth and life just happened.

She buzzed me to come to her room; she was pushing. I could see the first baby's head nearing her perineum. I asked one of the midwives to call the doctors to inform them that the twin birth was imminent. I prepared to receive the first baby. No one came. Where were they? It was 8:15 am, and they were at their daily morning staff meeting. They were called a second and third time, but no one arrived.

The pediatrician did arrive, and one midwife came in to help out. Both of those babies were born quickly and easily, one after the other, before the staff meeting was even over and before any other doctors arrived, before any medications were given, before any medical procedures were performed. It was quiet, the lights were low and there were no onlookers.

When the doctors did arrive, they found her upright in bed, cradling and breastfeeding two babies, smiling from ear to ear. I love it when women get what they want.

Lessons learned:

1. A determined woman who knows what she wants will collect like-minded people along the way who will support her on her path.
2. We empower one another. Her victory became my victory.
3. Nature knows what it is doing most of the time. There is an innate, natural wisdom and logic in birth, even with twins.
4. What needs to happen happens, though we did try to summon the doctors three times.

Nila

Avishag is a good friend of mine. She birthed all three of her babies with me. Her oldest, Nila, was born at the hospital while I was still working there, and the younger two were born at home. I have known her entire family since she was about ten years old.

Avishag became pregnant with Nila while she was living in Australia. She was a young woman living in the wild land of eucalyptus trees, parrots, koalas and kangaroos. She learned all about natural parenting and natural birth from the families in the community in which she lived. She dreamt of giving birth in her tent or joining the baby's father Ze'ev in India and having the baby there. She even met with a local home birth midwife who was so laid back that she didn't even ask her to do even one organ scan.

But Chana, her mother in Israel, felt differently about things and over the phone begged her to do some testing. She gave in to her mother's request and did one organ scan which was normal, but for Avishag it felt unnecessary because she felt wonderful and she was confident that everything was okay.

While visiting a friend before she left Australia, she met a woman who turned out to be a midwife, who noticed that she was pregnant, approached her and gave her the book *Hearts Open Wide: Midwives and Births,* a book about home birth in California. It was filled with inspiring stories and photographs. She asked her to pass the book on to a midwife when she returned to Israel, so in the middle of her eighth month, when she decided to come home to Israel, she looked for the woman who would receive the book. She didn't know any midwives in Israel, but Chana who knew her like every mother knows her daughter understood what she needed and suggested that she contact me.

Ze'ev returned to Israel in early August after falling off a cliff in India. They both did a quick birth preparation course with me, and together we decided that I would deliver their baby at the hospital and that I would come in even if I was not on shift.

Everything in Israel seemed strange and foreign to Avishag. She had returned from the dead of winter in Australia to the oppressive heat of the Israeli summer. Demands were made of her to supplement the minimal prenatal care she had received with additional blood and urine tests and more organ scans. I tried to manage her opposition, to help her to find the middle ground and to provide a voice of reason and compromise.

Close to her due date, Ze'ev became very ill, and his condition deteriorated quickly. At first, no one knew what was wrong with him. He was hospitalized in the intensive care unit. Avishag was frantic. Eventually the doctors discovered that the cause of the disease was Salmonella. He received buckets of intravenous antibiotics and made a full recovery.

Two days after he was released from the hospital, Avishag was 42 weeks gestation, and there were no signs of impending labor. She went to the hospital with Ze'ev and Chana for a post-date check-up. She was told that everything concerning the baby looked fine and that her estimated weight was 3.000 kg. They left the hospital relieved and happy and celebrated with a meal in the nearby Druze village, Daliyat al Carmel.

They went home, went to bed, slept until late the next morning and then napped again in the afternoon. Then a strong contraction woke Avishag up from her nap and got her out of bed. She walked around the yard with contractions all afternoon and evening, while friends visited with her and Ze'ev. In addition, because her younger brother, Yiftach, was celebrating his 12th birthday, the house was filled with friends, balloons, gifts, food and birthday cake. It was a bit hectic; Yiftach was concerned that for the rest of his life he might have to share his birthday with his niece.

Later in the evening, the contractions began to get stronger and more frequent, but Avishag still felt comfortable at home, mostly in the bathtub. When the contractions started coming every four minutes she realized that it was time to start moving in the direction of the delivery room. They got into the car, together with Chana and Ze'ev's brother, Adam. Avishag took her pillow with her.

They arrived at the hospital around 11 pm. Avishag was wearing a colorful, quilted vintage dress from the 1970s. Ze' ev, in all his glory, was barefoot with dreadlocks down to his waist, wearing an ethnic vest on his hairy, bare chest and a tie-dyed lungi wrapped around his waist. The midwives and doctors on the shift were taken aback by their appearances. Ze'ev looked like a caveman to them.

Avishag's cervix was dilated seven centimeters. She took off the dress and walked through the hallway naked, not because she was bold, but because it felt natural and comfortable. She took a nice, long shower and refused all other forms of pain relief. They asked for me, but I wasn't working.

I was at a wedding when I received the telephone call. My son Eitan received a call from Avishag's brother, Yoav. He was begging me to go to the hospital to help Avishag. She was in a bit of a pickle. She was refusing fetal monitoring, refusing an IV line and refusing just about anything and everything else they wanted to give her or do to her. The staff didn't know how to handle the situation, and they were refusing to take care of her as long as she kept refusing to receive their care. They had hit an impasse.

I quickly went home, changed my clothes and drove to the hospital. When I entered the delivery suite everyone sighed a deep sigh of relief because this couple was the farthest from the average hospital patients that they had encountered. Avishag was naked, on her hands and knees, moaning and swaying. The room was dark and ethnic music was playing in the background. Ze'ev was standing by the bed, a caveman among the machines.

They were thrilled to see me, someone who could understand what they wanted – just to give birth, with no interventions or drugs. Later they told me that as I entered the room, they imagined hearing the theme song from *Superman* and could envision my red cape and a big S on my chest. I was there to save the day. I was their breath of fresh air.

We sorted out the bureaucracy with the doctor on call. Avishag signed forms stating that she was refusing standard obstetric care, and then they left us alone. We closed the door, created a safe space and got on with the business of birthing this baby.

Less than an hour later at 1:22, Nila was born, beautiful and robust, screaming her head off so that everyone could hear that she was perfectly fine. I wiped her off and handed her to her mother. She found her place on Avishag's chest, got comfortable and stayed there for a long, long time. I went to find Chana, the new grandmother, so that she could come meet baby Nila.

Avishag and Nila had danced the dance of labor without the fetal monitor, without drugs and without anyone's help. They did it their way, naked among the machines, with their hearts wide open. I was honored to be a part of this wild birth even though it took place in captivity. Avishag and Ze'ev taught me how important it is to hold on to the dream, to be true to oneself, even when the burden of conformity presses in from all directions.

And Yiftach was so happy that Nila got her own birthday.

Avishag and I continued to cross paths. She became a childbirth education teacher and a lactation consultant. She recommended me to many of her friends whose babies I delivered at home and at my birth center. She was with us at many of those births.

Her next two births were at home; the first was in the tent that she, Ze'ev and Nila were living in, and the second in a kiddie pool in the garden. At Avishag's 40th birthday party, she was surrounded by good friends, and among them were almost 30 children whose entrance into the world I had witnessed, Nila being the oldest in the tribe. She will always hold a special place in my heart.

Lessons learned:
1. Avishag and Ze'ev taught me to be true to myself, just as they had remained true to themselves. They held onto their dream and achieved it.
2. I felt a great sense of safety with this couple because of the responsibility they took for themselves and their decisions.
3. A home-like atmosphere can be created within the confines of the hospital. This birth planted the seeds in my mind of what was to come to fruition in the not-so-distant future; I was to become a home birth midwife.

The Truck and the Motorcycle

For several years I taught childbirth preparation classes at a community center in Yokneam Illit. At the time Yokneam was at the height of a huge expansion, and many young, professional couples relocated there from Haifa. Twice a week I had classes filled with couples having their first babies and becoming parents for the first time.

One of the women whose name I can't remember approached me for advice after class about a problem she had. She suffered from vaginismus that was so severe that she and her husband had never had intercourse. The baby they were expecting had been conceived via artificial insemination with his sperm.

I asked no questions about her past, but really wanted to help her get through this, and have a good birth experience. She had never been in therapy for this issue, and it created an understandable strain on their marital relationship. She wanted to give birth naturally without the help of any drugs. This made everything even more challenging. The usual approach to helping women with vaginismus to get through the birth is to give them an epidural as soon as possible. This creates a neural block for the lower half of the body and makes vaginal exams and pushing easier for everyone. A natural birth would not afford these advantages.

Luck, karma, serendipity, fate, synchronicity and the stars were all lined up on the day she came into the delivery room in active labor. I was working a morning shift, and it was a particularly quiet day. I took her on as my sole client during that shift, and invested a lot of time and effort into finding out how to help her through this challenge.

We closed the door; privacy was a must. She remained in her bra and underwear; walking around half naked was not a good feeling. I did not examine her vaginally at all and depended on other observable cues that indicated that the labor was progressing: her posture transforming from upright to horizontal, the tone of her voice going lower and deeper, the location of her pain moving forward from her lower abdomen into her pelvic floor and the urge to push appearing gradually as the head moved down.

She was deep inside herself, picking up on the same cues, feeling the baby's head move down through her pelvis. She laid on her side covered with a bedsheet throughout the entire pushing phase. I encouraged her without giving her instructions. I gave her positive feedback when I saw that she was progressing. She received lots of love and support from her partner. She was excited to experience herself as strong and capable, coping and succeeding.

And then it happened. She pushed her baby girl out, took her into her arms and wept. We were all filled with awe of her courage, her fortitude and her success. It was a moment I will never forget.

A few weeks later she called me to give me an update. She was riding high on her victory and came to some significant understandings about herself and what she was capable of. One of them was that she was ready to go into therapy in order to solve her problem for the sake of her marriage. Another was that after she had experienced a truck coming out of her vagina there should be no problem letting in a motorcycle.

With a huge grin on my face, I wished her the best of luck. The healing had already begun.

Lessons learned:
1. Without knowing whether or not she was a survivor of sexual violence I treated her as if she was. It was lucky for both of us that the labor room was quiet that day. This enabled me to provide her with all the time and patience that she needed. This isn't always possible in a public hospital, but it worked out perfectly for us.
2. I was in awe of this woman who knew exactly what she needed and went after her vision. I learned that in cases like this, fate has no choice but to cooperate.
3. Vaginismus is not a life sentence. A good, empowering birth can make all the difference.

Not According to the Plan

Noga was another woman who had participated in one of my birth preparation courses and then found herself in the delivery room with her husband Guy during one of my shifts. She was as happy to see me as I was to see her. I had developed an affinity for taking care of women whom I had gotten to know before they walked into the delivery room in the throes of labor. There was a basis for communication, something to build on during the birth. Taking care of strangers was satisfying, but taking care of women I knew was always a special treat.

Noga was a clinical psychologist. She stood out in her group as highly intelligent, well read and mature. She was also extremely motivated to experience a natural birth. She had carefully prepared a birth plan in which she clearly stated that she was not interested in receiving any pharmacological pain relief, being induced or having her labor fiddled with in any manner. These were some of my favorite women to take care of, women who were highly educated and highly motivated to achieve natural births. More cynical birth workers might say that these are the women who are most likely to end up with C-sections. Noga did not end up with a C-section, but she did experience almost everything else on the list of what she didn't want.

Noga's birth started before midnight, and she called me to let me know. I explained to her that I was going to bed and that I would be coming in for a morning shift in less than eight hours. If she could wait we would meet in the delivery room. If not I would come visit her and her baby in the postpartum ward.

When I came out of the elevator the first person I ran into was Guy. He told me that Noga's contractions had stalled and that there was very little progress. I got dressed, joined the morning shift and asked to be assigned to room seven where Noga and Guy were, hoping I could be their midwife. And so it was.

Noga's labor was long and exhausting. She agreed to have her membranes ruptured, hoping that this would move things along. It didn't really help, so the doctors recommended augmenting her labor with Pitocin and she agreed. The contractions were much more painful than she had anticipated, and she decided to ask for epidural anesthesia. This had not been her plan, but she still felt very much in control of her birth experience because she made all the decisions in cooperation with the doctors after consulting with me and Guy.

Noga's cervix was eventually fully dilated, and the baby's head started coming down. She pushed for hours until she couldn't push anymore. She asked to speak with the doctor on call, and together they decided to deliver the baby via vacuum delivery. With her permission he cut an episiotomy and brought her baby out of her body and into her waiting arms. She was ecstatic.

Even though things hadn't gone according to plan she had been a full participant in the decision-making process, had received all the information necessary in order to do so and she felt that she had been treated as an autonomous individual. This made all the difference in the world.

And as they say, "Man plans and God laughs." Noga immediately saw the irony inherent in the situation and still laughs at herself, her plans and how her birth turned out in the end. I was never worried that Noga would walk away from her birth feeling traumatized mainly because no one ever took away her power, and she had lots of time to absorb each situation as it presented itself. She asked questions, received answers, understood her options and made decisions concerning her body and her baby.

Lessons learned:
1. To a certain extent, women are able to impact when they will go into active labor, especially if it will determine who will be there to support them.
2. When birthing women are provided with information, and with enough time to understand and process it, birth interventions are not experienced as violent and aggressive but as helpful.
3. Autonomy and a sense of ownership of the body contribute to feelings of control and empowerment during birth. The outcome of Noga's birth was less important than the manner in which she experienced it.
4. Humor is a reassuring sign of good health and healing.

Just Like Her Cat

Ophir is a friend of my son Udi who recommended me to her for childbirth preparation. She wasn't really interested, but Udi was insistent. He had learned from me that women do better if they are prepared, that knowledge is power and that if you don't know your choices, you have no choices.

She and her husband remained reluctant, but a few days before her due date they decided to come. I paired them up with another couple who seemed to be in a similar mindset. The five of us spent two hours together mostly talking about how to achieve a satisfying birth experience in a hospital setting. Ofir confidently stated that she intended to give birth like her cat, simply and naturally.

Again, as fate would have it, I was working when Ophir arrived in the delivery room in active labor. She was the perfect candidate for the new natural birthing suite which had been open for just a few weeks. She was happy to take advantage of its facilities which included an ensuite bathtub, shower and toilet, which none of the other rooms had.

But she never actually used them. She spent most of the labor outside in the corridor with her family and friends, smoking cigarettes and just hanging out. It was impossible to know from her behavior how rapidly the labor was progressing, so every once in a while I fished her out of her huddle and brought her back in for a few minutes of fetal monitoring and a vaginal check. She was having strong contractions every three minutes, and her cervix was dilating at lightning speed.

At nine centimeters, I convinced her and her partner to accompany me back into the delivery room and get ready for the baby's arrival. Fifteen minutes later the baby was cooing in her arms. Ophir was relaxed and happy, and she smiled up at me from the bed. She really had given birth just like her cat, so simply, so naturally and so unburdened by worries, birth plans or unnecessary knowledge. Women know what they are capable of. This lesson keeps coming back to me.

A few years later when Ophir came back to the delivery room to deliver her second baby I wasn't working there anymore, but she did telephone me to tell me about the birth.

She woke up in the middle of the night with contractions. By the time she and her partner got to the delivery room it was between five and six am. She was six centimeters dilated and was in active labor. By the time all the paperwork was done and they got settled in the natural birthing suite, it was close to seven am when the shifts changed. The midwife who announced that she would be working with them was not to her liking at all. Ophir felt turned off by her and didn't feel comfortable with the idea of her delivering her baby.

Her contractions eased off gradually, getting farther and farther apart, less and less painful. By the time the doctors and midwives did rounds at 8:30, her contractions had disappeared completely both according to the monitor and according to her feeling. One of the doctors examined her and found that the baby's head was high, and her cervix was thick and dilated three centimeters. He declared that she wasn't in labor at all and sent her home. Ophir was happy because she didn't like the midwife anyway.

She returned to the delivery room a week and a half later and gave birth within an hour from the time she arrived at the hospital. Who was it who said that she gives birth like her cat?

Lessons learned:
1. The physical conditions that support progress in labor are vastly different from one woman to the next. Our job is to avoid judging the woman for her choices. I would not have chosen to hang out in the corridor and smoke cigarettes, but it wasn't my birth.
2. Some women have stronger defensive instincts when it comes to safety during labor. As long as Ophir felt safe and supported her labor flowed. As soon as she felt threatened it stopped. Something deep inside of her shouted "No!"
3. A lack of safety can trigger the cervix to close and cause the head to rise in the pelvis.
4. A midwife who comes to work with a sour look on her face can stop labor.
5. Our unconscious parts are much more influential on the labor process than our conscious parts.

Labor Positions

When I first learned to deliver babies all the women were in bed either lying on their sides during the first stage of labor or lying on their backs during the second stage. When pushing, their feet were either in stirrups or set up against them. I never saw a woman give birth in any other position. It was relatively convenient for me and provided a good view of the perineum and control over the situation. This was what I was taught and practiced, and this was what I taught my students. That was until my world was cracked open at a *Midwifery Today* Conference in London.

I went together with my friend Leslie. There we heard lectures, watched slide shows and listened to first-hand reports of women being upright and active during labor and giving birth squatting, standing, on hands and knees, on birthing stools and in birthing pools. It all made sense, taking gravity into account as a force in nature and water as a well-known source of comfort and healing.

Our minds were blown open. We would never be the same. We came home and made a 5-year plan for the changes we wanted to see happen in the delivery room. We started by going to visit Misgav Ladach, the only hospital in Israel that at the time promoted and supported natural birth. We wanted to see a water birth, to see women birthing in upright positions and we wanted to meet and talk with the midwives who were doing this work.

We spent two days at the delivery room, seeing things we had never seen. We came home a bit jealous but optimistic that we would be able to make changes in our own personal midwifery styles and in the general atmosphere in the delivery room. This was easier said than done, and the process was long and very gradual. Some of the changes were made unexpectedly and without any preparation. Some were made through the work of committees and the creation of protocols. Together this created the dawn of a new era in the delivery room, a window in the stone wall of tradition, habit and the routine practice of laying women down on their backs to give birth to their babies.

Knee-Chest Position

One morning shift I was caring for an Arab woman who spoke no Hebrew. This was her sixth delivery, and all of her previous births had been normal, quick and straightforward. But not this time. Something was keeping that baby from coming down, and the doctors began discussing taking her to a C-section. It seemed like such a shame, and I busted my brain trying to come up with a solution in order to dodge the surgical option for bringing this birth to its conclusion.

And then I remembered that I had heard about the use of the knees-chest position in order to turn persistent occipito-posterior positions (POPP), a situation that makes births longer and more difficult for the baby to come down and out because the head is positioned in an unusual way. I felt that I needed permission from my supervisor to do something so seemingly radical at the time. I told Rina of my idea, explained how it should work and convinced her to let me try. I went back into the room and saw this woman lying in the bed, groaning with each contraction and trying desperately to push out her baby, who wasn't cooperating. We had no common language, and it was going to be a challenge to get her to flip over.

I used pantomime and hand gestures to try and relay the message but eventually got down on the floor and showed her what I wanted her to do. She reluctantly made the move and got into a knees-chest position. I could sense that this was terribly uncomfortable for her because she was upside down, her butt was in the air and it was difficult for her to breathe. I was afraid she would turn right back over, so I breathed together with her with my face close to hers. She managed to breathe through five contractions and then flipped over on her back. The next contraction was strong and long, and without any warning whatsoever, she pushed the baby out and I caught it in my bare hands. There wasn't even time for gloves.

Needless to say, this was a glorious success, and the news spread quickly through the delivery room. Everyone wanted to understand what we did and how it could be of use in other challenging situations. Within a few months, any time a baby was stuck and wasn't coming out, the question that began to be asked by the doctors was: "Did you try knees-chest?" It was a small but significant victory.

Lessons Learned:

1. It is worthwhile to learn from the experience and wisdom of midwives all over the world and put that wisdom into practice.
2. It is worthwhile to try new things, even though they will not be considered acceptable at first.
3. Good will and an open heart are enough to get through the barrier of language.
4. In order to move the baby, move the mother.

On All Fours

My next experience with an alternative birthing position was during an evening shift with a very full delivery room. All the beds were occupied, including those that were usually reserved for women not in active labor. One of the women under my care was progressing more quickly than anyone anticipated, and each time I checked her she appeared to be deeper and deeper inside herself, coping with more and more intense contractions.

I started preparing to receive the baby, and she caught what I was doing out of the corner of her eye. Through a fog of birth hormones, she told me that she wanted to give birth like her dog. I asked her, "And how does your dog give birth?" Her answer was plain and simple, "On all fours."

I was surprised, shocked and really excited all at once. I had never delivered a baby with the mother pushing on her hands and knees. I admitted to her that I had no experience with this, but I would try to do my best. She assured me that I would be just fine.

Before I could gather my thoughts and prepare myself in any way, she started pushing, and her perineum was beginning to bulge. Everything was upside down. I wasn't sure where to place my hands or how to protect her from tearing. Which was the first shoulder now and which would be the second shoulder?

I didn't have much time for deliberation because within seconds the baby slipped out and into my hands with the help of the next contraction. The baby was in my hands, the mother acrobatically raised her leg over the cord, took him to her chest and looked up at me and smiled, "I told you everything would be okay."

When I got home, I couldn't sleep. I searched through all my textbooks trying to understand the physiological mechanism of the birth of the shoulders. I had been taught that the anterior shoulder was the first to exit, but in this birth the posterior shoulder came out first.

I had witnessed something new. I tried to understand why I had been taught the opposite. I remembered that the basis for midwifery learning during the last 200 years has all been based on women lying on their backs. When women rise up and get off of their backs, birth looks different.

Lessons Learned:

1. I am a lot less important than I thought when it comes to preventing tears. I didn't have the time to protect her perineum with my hands, and nothing horrible happened. The baby slipped right out and left no marks.
2. When the birthing woman is relaxed and happy, so is her pelvic floor. In this case, it simply opened itself up and invited the baby to arrive.
3. A self-confident woman can impart a lot of confidence in her midwife. This woman believed in me and by doing so, enabled me to believe in myself just a little bit more.

Standing Up for Herself

One Friday evening I was washing dishes after dinner with my family. Both my sons, who were soldiers at the time, were out for the evening with their friends, each with one of our two cars.

I received a phone call from the delivery room. There was a woman there named Michal who refused to lay down in bed, wouldn't get out of the shower, and declared that she intended to give birth to her baby standing up.

Michal had been in touch with me during her pregnancy along with several other midwives. She was trying to find the right place to have a corrective birth experience. Her first birth had been disempowering and a negative encounter with the medical establishment. She was also considering giving birth at home. We had talked a few times, but never met.

The midwife on the phone asked if I could come in to deliver this woman. There was both panic and urgency in her voice. There was no way I could explain to her what to do over the phone. I told her I was willing to come in, but I had no car. Then I heard Michal's husband who was hovering nearby say that he would gladly come pick me up. I agreed.

On the way to the hospital, I learned as much as possible from her husband as I could. Some of what he told me I already knew. This was Michal's second birth; the first had been traumatic. She was in search of a corrective experience and was determined not to relinquish control to the doctors and midwives. She wanted to do it her way this time and hopefully regain her sense of control over her body and her life.

I arrived and found her in the shower groaning. She sounded very close to full dilation, and this was confirmed when I examined her while she was standing in the shower. She wanted to fill me in on all the details of her birth plan, but I assured her that there was no need and that I would do whatever she asked.

I gently urged her to come with me to the delivery room, and I promised her that we would find a way to birth this baby without her lying down in a bed. She put on her bathrobe, and together we slowly made our way over to the birthing room. She stood next to the bed and leaned on it during the contractions. In between, I gathered towels and sheets, stood behind her and prepared for the arrival of the baby. She was howling, and I could hear in her voice that she was in charge. It was the sound of a woman in her power.

I couldn't see anything, but I could feel the head pressing down into the palm of my hand through her perineum. I sat down on the chair behind her, supporting the baby's head, and then he just slipped into my hands. She reached down and took him to her chest; I got up off the chair, and she sat down where I had been with her baby secure in her arms. It was that simple.

A few minutes later the placenta came out, and she and her baby got cleaned up and into the bed together. Maybe half an hour had passed since the moment I arrived at the hospital. The midwives were curious and wanted to come in. They asked politely if I needed any help.

I stayed a few more minutes but was anxious to get home, so I let them clean up, write up the birth and do the postpartum care. I took a taxi home. It felt historic.

The next day I worked an evening shift with the same midwife who had called me in such a panic the evening before. She asked me to show her how I had delivered a baby with the woman standing up. I was happy to demonstrate and explain, but the situation was a bit awkward for me because she had 30 years more experience as a midwife than I had. But if she was willing to learn, I was willing to teach. She was also the same midwife who told me that I had more luck than brains.

We went into the same room and next to the same bed, and with the same chair I showed her exactly what I had done. Her reaction was priceless. She looked at me and said, "It's so simple. I could have done that." I agreed. Yes, it was so simple, and yes, she could have done it.

We can all learn lots of new things if we are not afraid to change.

Lessons learned:
1. A woman who suffered a traumatic birth and is seeking a healing experience is like a force of Nature; she can't be stopped. It is preferable to join forces with her and avoid standing in her way. She is going to get the birth she needs.
2. A standing birth is just like a birth on hands and knees but without the bed. It is a good idea to prepare and use lots of towels and pillows if they are available. The floor is quite a distance away.
3. I love challenges; I love learning new things. I embrace change. I enjoy sharing my knowledge with other midwives.
4. The fear of change keeps us stuck in time. Avoiding change prevents us from growing and evolving. It is worthwhile to see change as an opportunity and not as a threat.

Closed Legs

One day, I had in my care a very young Arabic-speaking woman in her third pregnancy. She had a lot of difficulty exposing her body and being examined; she barely spoke Hebrew, but somehow she managed to communicate to me both her difficulties and her needs. She wanted to be covered with the sheet at all times and she clearly wanted her husband and mother-in-law out of the room.

During most of the birth she laid on her side breathing and groaning through the contractions. It was difficult to hear the progress she was making because there was very little modulation in the volume or tone of her voice. I sensed that she was entering the transition phase of labor when she added a subtle pushing effort at the end of each contraction and seemed a bit agitated.

I gathered all the equipment I needed for the delivery and sat by her on a chair and waited together with her, one contraction at a time. She was lying on her side with her legs tightly pressed together and covered with the sheet up to her eyes. I offered to hold her hand and massage her back, but she clearly wasn't interested. I peeked under the sheet and saw that her perineum was beginning to bulge. I tried to encourage her to lie on her back for the delivery, but her resistance was uncompromising. I tried to hold up her upper leg so that she could deliver side-lying. No luck. She went back to the way she was with her legs tightly closed together.

I felt myself entering unknown territory. I had never encountered a woman who so emphatically resisted opening her legs to deliver her baby, but I wanted to respect her need and not violate her trust. My feeling was that she had been violated before. She continued to quietly push, and I continued to peek under the sheet every once in a while at her bulging perineum. There was no coaching, no discussions, no feedback, no right or wrong. There was just one woman lying on her side, pushing a baby out, and another woman, sitting by her side and waiting.

And then it happened. The baby's head slipped out, and her legs were still tightly pressed together! I had never seen anything like this before. It was shocking to see the baby's head tucked between her butt and her thighs. I gently asked permission to open one knee in order to let the rest of the body out. It was an automatic reaction. I had seen the head come out, but I was wary about the shoulders. For a split second she opened one knee, and I slipped the shoulders out. She immediately closed her legs again, took the baby into her arms and covered herself again.

I could tell by the look in her eyes that she was thankful for the respect I had paid to her needs. I am still eternally grateful to her for the valuable lesson she taught me; women don't need to open their legs in order to push their babies out.

Lessons learned:
1. When a woman shows signs that her body has been violated, she doesn't need to tell her story in order to receive appropriate trauma-sensitive care which includes: few or no vaginal exams, protection of her privacy and modesty, recognition of her pain and difficulty, affirmation of her requests and emotional support without the aid of words.
2. There is no need to ask questions or to hear the story.
3. It is possible to deeply understand what a woman needs without verbal communication with her.
4. There is something exciting and moving about letting go of control and allowing the birthing woman to lead the way. It is like getting on a train without knowing the destination. Otherwise, how would I have learned that women don't need to spread their legs wide open in order to birth their babies?

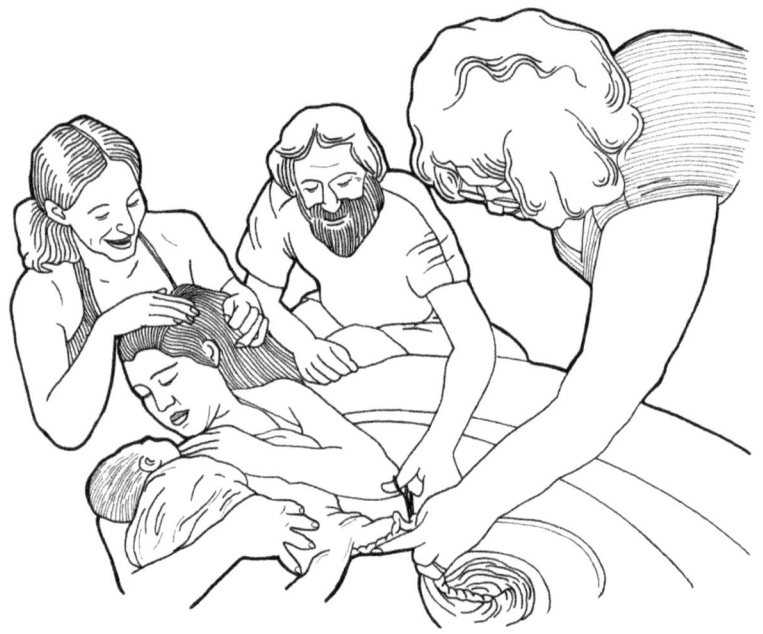

Women are Capable of Anything – Births at Home

Leaving the delivery room and launching a new career as a home birth midwife was one of the easiest decisions I have ever made. There was no effort, no making lists of pros and cons, no sleepless nights staring at the ceiling trying to decide. It was like an apple that didn't even need to be plucked off the tree; I just held my hand under it, and it dropped right into my hand like an easy birth.

When I notified Rina, my supervisor, of my decision, I expected her reaction to be one of either anger or disappointment. Instead, she surprised me by smiling at me and asking, "What took you so long?" She knew in her heart of hearts that I was in her delivery room temporarily and actually on a path to practicing independently as a home birth midwife.

I had been reading books and researching the topic for years, knowing that someday this moment would arrive. Finally, the time had come to create my own home birth business. I needed to purchase and organize equipment, create forms, gather phone numbers, buy insurance and get as much advice as possible from the veteran home birth midwives who were already doing this work.

Saying Yes from Now On

A few weeks before I made the decision to leave the hospital, I gave a talk about empowerment in birth at a conference for pregnant women. After my lecture and during the break, a beautiful young woman named Lior approached me. She was wearing a huge smile on her face, a long, flowing skirt and a flower in her beautiful black hair. She asked me to be her midwife and deliver her baby at home. I was a bit stunned because I was still working in the hospital, and I answered her, "I don't do home births." She didn't blink an eye before she laughed and answered me right back, "You do now."

Lior and her husband Nati had recently arrived in Israel after living in New Zealand for a few years. There for her first pregnancy, she chose to do her prenatal care with a midwife and to give birth at home, an option supported by the national medical system. She was convinced that I could do this too; intuitively, she felt that I was the right person for the job and she helped me decide to cut my cord to the delivery room.

We met several times, got to know one another gradually and formed the kind of midwife-client relationship that I had only read about in books. She seemed to be a very strong and determined woman. Because she had experienced one more home birth than I had, I learned from her. Her first birth had ended up in a transfer to the hospital and a vacuum-assisted delivery that was a bit traumatic for her. This time she wanted to push her baby into the world at home under her own steam.

It was the eve of Succoth, and Lior was in week 39 feeling healthy, happy, and excited to become the mother of two sweet little girls. We talked that morning, and she complained about some swelling in her legs and feet. I suggested a possible connection between swelling and stuck emotions and asked if that touched her in any way. She promised to give it some thought. She called me again at 1 pm with contractions; her waters had broken a few minutes before. She seemed to have gotten those emotions moving.

I was in the middle of making spicy fish and couscous for our holiday dinner. On the phone, Lior sounded very serious, concentrated and quiet. She was alone in bed with her napping daughter and was waiting for Nati to arrive from work. My first instinct was to rush off and leave the food on the stove, but I decided that finishing the preparation would take only a few minutes, so I did.

I got ready, packed my bags into the car, kissed Avner goodbye, told him to wish me good luck and drove off to Haifa. It was only my first home birth, and I would already be missing a holiday dinner with my family.

I called my midwife friend Tia on the way to share my excitement and get some words of wisdom. She heard me out and wished me good luck. She hinted that, in her opinion, I shouldn't be alone. Maya had been planning to be with me as the second midwife at this birth, but as luck would have it, she was in the Negev with her family, and I would have to go it alone.

I arrived a little before 2 pm and found Lior and Nati in the living room of their bare and spotlessly clean garden apartment. Despite the date, it was unseasonably hot; luckily the living room had thick walls and was relatively cool. All the windows were wide open. Lior was on her knees leaning on a small coffee table which she had turned into an altar of sorts. She had a cup with water and orange oil to smell and spread on her lips, Rescue Remedy for raised anxiety levels, water to drink and a pillow to lean on. She was clearly in active labor and was handling it well. I sat on the couch and soaked in the atmosphere. Nati was a little uneasy and was trying to figure out what to do with himself. Lior wanted him to be with her, and he wanted to be just about anywhere else. Luckily for him, their baby girl Yahel woke up, and Nati was asked to take her to the neighbors.

I listened to the baby's heartbeat which was fine. Lior asked me to examine her. I found that her cervix was six centimeters dilated, 100% effaced, and the head was at S-1. Great!

Her labor gradually got more intense. She had moments that were difficult for her. She held on tightly to the table and bit Nati once or twice. She even let out a scream here and there. I massaged her back with oil according to her instructions and pressed her hip bones during the contractions. I felt like she wanted to be mothered. She was not interested in either a bath or a shower.

At about 3:30 she apologized and gave a long speech about how she couldn't handle it anymore and how she wanted to go to the hospital for an epidural. I heard her out to the end and asked her if she wanted to be examined. She said yes, and to the delight of all of us, she was fully dilated, the head was at S+1. She wasn't pushing yet but was happy to hear the news, even though it was difficult for her to believe that it was really true.

A few contractions later, she started pushing and had difficulty relaxing her pelvic floor. Eventually, she figured out how to open up, and she gave it her all. She started pushing with all her heart and soul, doing splits on the floor. The baby was born at 4 pm on the button, and Lior was still in the same position she had been for two hours leaning on the coffee table. She tore as the baby was born. The baby weighed a whopping 4.2 kg. There was some difficulty getting the shoulders out. I tried one shoulder, then the other, and the first shoulder again, and then she came loose, presenting with the chubby cheeks of a month-old baby. We were all relieved, happy to welcome the baby and sweating profusely.

A few minutes later there was a slight gush of blood and a few cramps, and it seemed like the placenta was on its way out, but this was only partially true. Lior gave a good push, and the placenta slid out into my gloved hand but not in its entirety. Part of it was still stuck inside, and nothing I did helped the placenta to separate from the wall of Lior's womb. Something was stubbornly pulling on it from inside.

It was so hot that my glasses steamed up, and the sweat stung my eyes. Lior's blood pressure and pulse were normal, and she wasn't bleeding, but the placenta was not coming out. Tia just happened to call to find out how things were going, and I told her what was happening. She suggested that I do all the things I had already done, but it was good to hear her voice. She also suggested I put in an IV line, but after I called the ambulance and understood how close the station was and how quickly they would arrive, I decided that the time could be better spent getting Lior dressed and ready for the transfer. She still wasn't bleeding.

The ambulance came almost immediately; the station was literally right down the road. Lior was feeling a little weak but okay for a woman who had just pushed out a 4.2 kg. baby. She hadn't packed a bag, so we gathered together her documents, her identity card and a few personal items. The crew decided to move her over to the ambulance without taking the time to put in an IV line. She drank water all the way to the hospital.

I called the delivery room to tell them that we were on our way. I cuddled the baby with the amazing cheeks in my arms. We all rode together in the ambulance. We were calm, Lior felt fine, and the baby was good. I had done the right thing and I knew it, even though it felt ominous. It was my first home birth, and here I was transferring. Was I being tested?

We arrived in the delivery room. My good friend Leslie and three other lovely midwives were working the evening shift. They were wonderful. Lior was put into room number four under Ruhama's charge. She tried to push on her belly a few times. The doctor on call did the same with more force, and eventually he managed to force the placenta out. It was white and ragged. She needed a manual revision of the uterine cavity under general anesthesia.

I had prepared Lior for this possibility, and she cooperated willingly. She understood that this had to be done. A big chunk of placenta came out, further justifying the transfer, the concern and the actions taken. This was a crazy way to start a new career, but there was a lot to be learned and a lot to be thankful for.

Lior perked up quickly and felt even better after a cup of the cinnamon apple tea that I had brought to the staff the day before as part of my going-away gift. We brought the baby back to her mama;

she nursed her and re-centered herself slowly. After much deliberation, she decided to spend the night at the hospital to be on the safe side.

Nati and I left the hospital at 9 pm, getting a ride back to the house from one of the neighbors. On the way home, I called Lihi, a home birth midwife and friend, to share the story with her. She was excited about the birth and couldn't believe the part about the transfer. I hadn't digested it either.

Lior chose to center her attention on the birth of the baby and not on the birth of the placenta. She focused on her success. Her objective had been to deliver her baby at home, on her own power, on her own terms, and she had achieved that goal. As far as she was concerned, the placenta was a minor detail.

This was an ironic and inglorious beginning. My transfer rate for home births would grow to become 14 percent. Transferring my first home birth to the delivery room that I had left a few days before was not only a statistical disaster, but it was also both embarrassing and humbling.

In time, I grew to become thankful for the medical assistance I would receive from hospitals when it was necessary. I also became wary of the trauma-ignorant culture of the delivery room, now witnessing it from a new perspective with the eyes and ears of an outsider. I was shocked to hear the harsh words, the threats and the lies that some women were exposed to. I was saddened to see the fatigue, the apathy and the lack of warmth that I sometimes witnessed among the midwives and doctors.

On the other hand, I was often pleasantly surprised by the flexibility, willingness to help and creativity that was showered upon us. My point of view gradually changed, as I moved forward into uncharted territory. I began to see things I hadn't seen when I was a part of the team. My blinders had been lifted.

Lessons learned:
1. Hands-and-knees position is great for contractions and pushing, but it doesn't give me enough control on the delivery especially if the baby is big. Side-lying for the final stage may be preferable in order to avoid tears. I didn't feel ready to suture yet, although some day I will.
2. I prefer an additional midwife to be with me at all births. This would be helpful if there is a problem and totally unnecessary if everything is fine. Better safe than sorry. Always.
3. I need to put some items in my backpack to have with me if I need to transfer: homeopathic Arnica, Bach Rescue Remedy, and transfer forms.
4. The woman should prepare a bag for the hospital ahead of time. From the time the ambulance is called, time flies and there is not enough time to start packing a bag.
5. I need to take my estimate of the fetal weight more seriously. At our last meeting I felt that the baby was big, but I erroneously put more emphasis on the estimate done at the hospital by the doctor than on my intuition, experience and knowledge.
6. A lot of amniotic fluid comes out with the baby. Many pads and towels on the floor are a good idea when the baby is on the way. I got soaked and so did the floor. The birth scene could have been cleaner.

A Single Mom and a New Pool

My second home birth was with Limor, a single mother with a five-year-old son named Or. She decided that it was time for another child and did what she needed to do in order to become inseminated by donor sperm. She lives together with her son in a house that she built on land given to her by her grandmother in an agricultural community. We came to know each other through Avishag.

On the morning of October 7, I woke up thinking about how often Limor had mentioned her love of the ocean. She had been at the beach several times in the last few weeks, hoping it would somehow bring on her labor. While relaxing during a Shiatsu treatment, it suddenly became clear that I needed to purchase all the equipment necessary for a water birth. Limor and I had discussed the possibility, but she felt unable to deal with the logistics and didn't have anyone who could take on the task. I decided to take responsibility.

That afternoon, with the pool, pump and hose in hand, I went to Limor's house to do a dry run on the equipment. Avishag and I made a date to meet there at 4:30 pm, but neither of us arrived on time. When we got there, we found Limor with her son and his cousin playing on the living room floor. Everything was as normal as could be. We listened to music, drank tea and talked.

Limor felt a contraction that literally came out of nowhere and after a few minutes another one. She went on about her business but had one eye on the oven clock in the kitchen. The contractions started coming closer to one another until we all realized that she was going into labor right there, in front of our eyes. I was both surprised and not. After all, the players were on the stage, and it was fitting that the performance should begin. On the other hand, I had never witnessed this kind of "induction" before. Her sister, Inbal, arrived from next door, and her friend Yael arrived from Tel Aviv. An impressive team of women had gathered together in order to support Limor through this auspicious event.

The contractions were coming three minutes apart and were not very painful. She was handling them well on her own by bouncing on the physio ball and being massaged by Yael. She paced around the house. We made sweet potato soup, Limor took a cake out of the freezer and we put lavender oil in the diffuser. The house smelled right for Limor who knew exactly what she wanted. We listened to music; Limor was the DJ, picking the CDs according to her shifting moods and needs.

The labor got more intense, and we filled the pool. The water was too hot, and we got busy cooling her off, bringing her ice cubes to suck on and wiping her brow. I think the warm water actually accelerated the pace of her labor. She got up to go to the bathroom, and on the way back to the pool, her waters broke. She got back into the pool, and the contractions became more intense. At one point she got out and sat on the ball again. She got tired and wanted to rest, so she went to lie down on the bed.

There she felt pressure and started to push. I assumed that she was fully dilated. There were trickles of blood coming intermittently. After about 20 minutes of pushing with no apparent progress, I checked her and it turned out that her cervix was still thick, only eight centimeters dilated and the head was still high. I broke out in a sweat. My thoughts raced in a thousand directions, and I was afraid that this birth, too, would end up in the hospital, maybe even with a C-section. I asked myself why the head was so high, why it wasn't coming down. Was I was being tested again?

My intuition kicked in. I understood that we had to get out of the room, off the bed, out of ready-for-the-baby mode and get back into dealing with contractions and the intense work of labor. I felt that Limor needed for a few things to happen in order to bring the head down: to cry or otherwise emote in a real way, to let go of her need for control and to get back into the water in order to ease her pain and recover her flow.

Limor didn't like learning that she was not about to give birth. It was taking more time than she had planned. The sun started to rise, and the dark blue light of dawn entered the room. She had planned to give birth during the night. Her sister Inbal and her friend Yael wore worried faces. I think they had moments when they doubted Limor's ability to give birth at home and my ability to watch over her safely and responsibly.

She had a few very intense moments in the bedroom when she suddenly found herself sprawled on the floor crying. Across from the bed on the wall, I noticed a photograph of her former boyfriend, the love of her life, who was killed in an automobile accident. Eventually she got back into the pool, then into the shower and gathered herself together. I examined her and she was fully dilated with the head at station +2. Thank God and the Goddesses! She did it.

Pushing was difficult at first, and Limor begged me to pull the baby out. When she understood that she had to push the baby out by herself, she did, and the baby was born at 6:06. The chorus of women around her pushed together with her, making guttural sounds that got higher pitched with each contraction and the subsequent progress of the head. By the time the baby was born, everyone was crying. What a night!

After the placenta came out, Limor separated the cord and put "Chamoud" (Cutie) to the breast. He was only interested in the right side. We cleaned up and got her comfortable. Everything was fine. The baby weighed approximately 2.6-2.7 kg (I didn't have an accurate scale at the time). He was skinny and long with surprisingly big hands and feet. He opened his eyes and looked around at the circle of women who had accompanied him into the world.

Limor showered, and we straightened up the house. Yael made tea, and we all laid down together in Limor's bed, helping her to come up with a name. The pediatrician came at 10:30 to examine the baby. He received a complete exam and a clean bill of health. She seemed surprised at the clean and relaxed atmosphere. Perhaps she was expecting to see blood smeared on the walls. I think we made a good impression.

We emptied and cleaned the pool; I packed my stuff and went home. Yael stayed with Limor and the baby. I didn't feel the lack of sleep; I was flying high on Limor's birth, stunned by those 45 difficult minutes and wondering what had kept the head up and what had brought it down in the end. I couldn't help but think that it had something to do with the man in the picture on the wall in the bedroom.

She named the baby Ma'ayan, which in Hebrew means "a spring," a natural source of flowing water.

Lessons learned:

1. Not to be lazy when there is no man around to do the technical work. Women can do anything.
2. The human environment has a powerful effect on the hormonal balance during the onset of labor. Limor was not in labor when we arrived and clearly went into active labor in the safety of our presence.
3. Childbirth should flow. If the flow stops, the process stops. Flow has many forms: in the breath, in movement, in thoughts and in emotions. One flow activates the other. It is important to pay attention to blockages.
4. At birth, something has to die before something else is born. Sometimes the woman giving birth needs to fall apart before she can be recreated.
5. There is no challenge that a circle of powerful women can't conquer.

Pushing on One Leg

My first encounter with Sigal was when I was lecturing at a doula course. When she called me a few months later, I didn't immediately remember her. Then we met and when I saw her face, I recalled the conversation we had had during the lunch break. I remembered her as older, quieter and more mature than most of the other doula students. She was interested in birthing at home and wanted to tell me her story.

Our first meeting was at my birth center without her husband. Sigal was 39 years old, and her daughter was six. She had experienced two ectopic pregnancies, two abortions and a miscarriage in addition to the birth of her daughter. The current pregnancy was the product of fertility treatments.

She described her first birth as traumatic; her needs had been ignored. She felt neither seen nor heard by any of the people who were supposed to support her. This time around she was determined to have a positive and corrective birthing experience.

Shortly after her first birth, Sigal developed neurological symptoms and was diagnosed with Multiple Sclerosis. At the time we met, she was not taking any medication, but in the past she had been treated with Interferon B. I was unsure about whether or not MS was a contraindication for a homebirth but decided to take her on as a client, with the uncertainty regarding the place of birth as an inherent part of our connection. She was willing to do the same, and we started meeting on a regular basis. We worked at getting to know each other better and creating a trusting relationship.

Sigal was born with a congenital club foot, and she underwent multiple surgeries as a tiny baby. Her earlier infancy was clouded by these experiences together with the difficulties of being mothered by a woman with postpartum depression. She yearned for a birth experience that would empower her and enable her to feel good about herself. She wanted to give birth in peace and quiet; she thought that birthing at home would be the key.

Eventually I met her partner, Jeremy, who seemed hesitant about a home birth but was trying to respect Sigal's wishes, but that changed. As the birth came closer, Sigal was more intent on birthing at home, and Jeremy wouldn't allow it to happen. At one of our meetings together, I began to feel that the home birth dilemma might be widening an already existing rift in their relationship. The differences between their lifestyles and approaches to life were obvious. He wanted to videotape the birth, and she was vehemently opposed to all forms of photography. This was only one example of the many issues they needed to resolve. Eventually Sigal chose to compromise, and we all agreed upon a birth that would start at home and would proceed to the hospital, with me acting as their doula. There was a plan.

Sigal's waters broke on a cold January morning at 4 am. Her contractions started at about 5:30 and they were coming fast and furious. I arrived at their house at about 6:30 am and found her with strong contractions every three minutes, dripping amniotic fluid and trying to get her daughter organized for school in between the waves. I watched her contractions become stronger and stronger. I examined her and found a cervical dilation of four centimeters. She was delighted with her progress and was very proud of herself. So was I.

By 7:40 she was literally crawling on the floor, vomiting intermittently and having a rough time. It was obvious that the time had come to get into the car and make our way to Poriya Hospital in Tiberias. Jeremy drove my car, and I sat with Sigal in the back seat. We listened to Indian meditation music, breathing together during contractions; Sigal closed her eyes and managed beautifully.

It was a gorgeous winter morning in the Galilee, and Jeremy drove us through fields of green all the way to the hospital. We were greeted by friendly faces, hugs and smiles and made a smooth transition into the delivery room. Sigal's Ob/Gyn, who also worked there, greeted us with his bright and shining smile. He was so happy that she had decided to give birth in the hospital and not at home.

The woman assigned to Sigal's care was Lynelle, a midwife from New Zealand, whom I had heard about but never met. She was an angel, sweet and soft-spoken and willing to let Sigal lead the way. Fetal monitoring was done standing up and on the birth ball. Sigal's cervix was six centimeters dilated, and she asked for an epidural. Lynelle put the IV line in, and the anesthesiologist arrived quickly.

Sigal was waging a battle inside herself, having dreamt and prepared for a natural birth, and here she was, in the delivery room with the anesthesiologist. He asked questions about what number of birth this was, how many centimeters dilated she was and how fast she was progressing. He promised to act according to her wishes, but he thought that the epidural was unnecessary. Sigal agreed and decided to let him go but made him promise to come back immediately if she changed her mind. He smiled, promised and left. She decided to try nitrous oxide (laughing gas).

She used the gas for a few minutes, but she was uncomfortable sitting upright. In an attempt to change positions, she put the mask aside for a few minutes, experienced a few contractions without the gas, realized that it was unnecessary, and pushed it away. She then stood up next to the bed, leaned on the birth ball and started swaying her hips and moaning. At 10:45 she was fully dilated.

When Sigal started pushing, her moans turned to groans and then to shouts. She was totally unselfconscious about her behavior, which for Sigal was revolutionary. She raised her right knee onto the bed, stood on the floor on her left foot and held on to Jeremy with her left hand and on to me with her right. Lynelle sat quietly behind her, coaching and supporting her all the time.

Sigal pushed in response to her own urges. Lynelle tried to encourage her to change position to something more stable and grounded, but I wagged my finger, signaling my disagreement, and nonverbally expressing my belief in Sigal's intuition. She was surely in this weird position for a reason, even though I didn't yet know what it was.

When the screaming turned into howling, I took advantage of a break in between pushes and whispered into Sigal's ear, reminding her that she wanted to push the baby out in a quiet, peaceful manner. She was silent for a moment while she digested what I had just said. She then took my suggestion to heart and started using "cloud breaths," a technique she had learned in her yoga class. Lynelle smiled and quietly said to her, "I don't know what you're doing, but keep doing it."

It felt right for Sigal too, and during the last two contractions, she breathed quietly and peacefully, and the baby tumbled out into Lynelle's gentle, waiting hands. He was big and beautiful, and his chubby little fist was clenched close to his cheek. Lynelle had held his elbow close to his chest to minimize potential damage to Sigal's soft tissues.

Lynelle helped Sigal onto the bed and placed the baby in her arms. She was overwhelmed with her feeling of accomplishment and cried out, "Wow, I gave birth to a boy!" It took days for her to digest the fact that she had really done it. Her husband was filled with respect, admiration and appreciation. No photographs, no videos, no machines. Just a very brave woman with a lot of support giving birth to a baby, standing on one leg! And she hadn't even torn. On the way home, I tried to digest some of what I had just witnessed.

I felt honored and privileged to accompany Sigal and be a part of her process. She victoriously achieved her goal, and everyone present enjoyed basking in the afterglow of her wisdom and her success. Empowerment is a truly contagious phenomenon.

Lessons learned:
1. Sigal saved her own perineum by raising her knee onto the bed. She did it because she felt her baby's elbow jamming into the right side of her birth canal. By pushing in this upright asymmetrical position, she relieved the pain, made room for the chubby little fist, and prevented a perineal tear. If she had been lying flat on her back, I shudder to think of what might have happened.
2. When women manage their own births they do amazing work, most of it highly intuitive.
3. Emotional support from loved ones and the solid presence of a wise midwife can go a long way in promoting a natural birth in a hospital setting. Empowering births can take place anywhere.
4. Corrective birth experiences happen. They can't be planned; the intention is the key. Ripples of healing undulate far and wide, affecting how we experience our past, our present and our future.

Doing it her Way

I first met Arij when she was in the 14th week of her second pregnancy. She was referred to me by Miriam Shibli from Nazareth Hospital after Arij mentioned to her that she wanted to give birth at home. I was delighted to meet Arij and her husband Nadim; they would turn out to be my first Arabic speaking clients.

They are both teachers who speak beautiful English. They had lived in the States and were extremely well informed about issues involving natural parenting, pregnancy and birth. Arij was anticipating her second birth after having a less than satisfying experience in a hospital in New York. A breastfeeding consultant there introduced them to natural parenting which eventually led them to the decision to give birth at home.

Dudu, their two-year-old son, was still actively nursing, and Arij was planning to continue nursing him through the pregnancy and the birth of the new baby. This opened up the world of tandem breastfeeding to me. I had never met a woman who breastfed a newborn while she was still nursing a two-year-old. Arij taught me a lot about this and about many other things during our acquaintance.

Arij was generally healthy and ate well despite her very skinny appearance. One of her sisters died in a fatal car accident, and Arij was still mourning her loss. In an organ scan at 23 weeks, there were some echogenic areas in the fetus' heart and bilaterally enlarged kidneys. Arij was confident that the baby was just fine and refused amniocentesis despite her doctor's insistence. This, along with her intention to birth at home and tandem breastfeed, created a rift between them. He was not used to dealing with such assertive, nonconformist and knowledgeable women.

Arij and Nadim moved to Jerusalem during the pregnancy but planned to give birth at Arij's mother's home in Nazareth. Arij described her mother as the original feminist, very well educated, free-spirited and free-thinking. At first her mother was apprehensive about the idea of a home birth but very quickly adjusted her attitude to accommodate her daughter's decision. She both respects and trusts Arij implicitly. A bedroom in her mother's home was designated as the birth room.

Arij had been GBS (Group B Streptococcus) positive in her first pregnancy and received antibiotics during the birth. This time she wanted to work to eradicate the GBS or if necessary, refuse antibiotic treatment. She used garlic slivers and sitz baths with grapefruit seed extract and was GBS negative when the vaginal swab was done. She was empowered by her success in eradicating the bacteria.

Arij's birth began with the breaking of her waters on January 31 at 12:45 pm while she was at the vegetable market in Nazareth. She hurried back to her mother's home after speaking to me on the phone. The contractions started building up gradually. I arrived at about 3:00, and her contractions were still sporadic. After about an hour they were coming every 3-5 minutes and were getting stronger. Dudu was nursing on and off, and the sucking clearly increased the frequency and intensity of Arij's uterine activity.

The birthing mama was hungry and had a large, nourishing lunch in between contractions. At 5 pm her cervix was seven centimeters dilated, and I called Maya, who was designated to be the second midwife. I knew Maya would enjoy being at this birth, so I called her relatively early. Dudu was still nursing on and off, and Arij still had the patience to be with him, to be sympathetic to his needs and to hold him in her arms while her uterus was pushing out his baby brother. She even managed to retain her sense of humor.

Eventually she felt herself losing her patience, handed Dudu over to her mother, and asked her to take him out of the house, to the home of her aunt, which was in the same complex. The birth really kicked in. Arij could now concentrate on herself and on coping with the increasingly painful and intense contractions. We turned down the lights in the bedroom, lit candles, played soft, soothing music and set the mood for Arij's home birth. A video camera arrived from one of Nadim's friends, and Maya happily became the official birth videographer.

The four of us had to manage to get around in this tiny room which was 80% occupied by a mattress on the floor. When it came time to push, we really felt the squeeze. Arij started pushing in a sitting position and then in a squat between the mattress and the closet but had more room and felt more comfortable lying on her side in the bed. Jude came into the world at 8:58 pm; everything was perfect and a bit surreal.

Arij's mother and Dudu heard Jude's first cries and came running up to the house even before the placenta was out. Dudu joined his new brother, shared his mother's chest with him and nursed, contracting his mother's uterus at the same time. Dudu was on the right breast, Jude on the left, Nadim supporting from behind and Arij laughing in the middle. Dudu was holding Jude's hand, and Maya captured it all on video.

Arij birthed exactly how she had planned, down to the smallest detail. Everything somehow fell into place. Dudu was with her, and even though he hadn't actually witnessed his brother as he came into the world, he surely understood that his mother had given birth at home. It was important to Arij and to Nadim to instill into the minds of their children that their parents did things their own way and that they could learn important lessons from that. Arij's mother had a rare opportunity to witness her daughter's perseverance and was as proud as a mother can be. Arij was tired but very happy, and she couldn't stop smiling. She imagined her OB's face after learning of her home birth, and her smile turned into a belly laugh.

Lessons learned:
1. I learned a lot about patience and respect for the intelligence and potential of small children. Arij trusted Dudu to lead the way in her mothering, and the process was fascinating to witness.
2. I encountered my judgmental self at about seven cm. when I was ready for Dudu to stop nursing, leave his mother alone and allow her to give birth to his brother. Arij eventually found the right time for her and for him, and it was long after the time I thought was right. I learn my best lessons when I'm wrong.
3. I learned a lot about one woman's personal struggle for independent thought and action. Arij was a true revolutionary. She received a lot of support from her mother and from her husband, and in many ways, Nadim was also a hero.
4. There is no one way to give birth at home. The options are infinite. Every birth looks, sounds, smells and tastes different.
5. A long prenatal period allows for a lot of time to get to know one another. We had ample time to grow to trust one another and make a connection.

Just A Few Hours Later

Just a few minutes after Jude was born, I received a phone call from Michal telling me that her labor had started. The contractions were still well spaced, but this was her second birth and anything could happen. I didn't hear from her again until I was in the car on my way home from Nazareth. The contractions were still far apart, but they were beginning to hurt and definitely weren't going away. Michal was 38+3 weeks and surprised that she was in labor so soon.

After I got home and relaxed, I told Avner all about Arij's birth and repacked my bags. I then received another call, this time from Michal's husband Ohad. When the partner calls it's because the mama can't talk. I felt the adrenaline surge through my body. I was surprisingly not concerned with the lack of sleep I was about to experience. I was just happy that the two women did not go into labor together and that they gave me a few hours of rest in between.

I arrived in Yodfat at 1:30 am. The house was clean and ready to greet the new baby. For Michal, it was her second birth, but for Ohad, it was his first. Michal had been briefly married to the father of her older son Tzuf. During her first birth, Michal labored basically on her own. It had been a difficult experience for her: an epidural, a long first stage, a hysterical second stage and an episiotomy. She was hopeful for an experience that would heal her wounds, and she had prepared emotionally and physically for this to happen. This time she hoped to be more present and aware.

Michal designs socks for Yodfat Textiles. Ohad is a farmer. They live in a big, new, beautifully designed and furnished house. One of the questions that was raised during the pregnancy was where in the house they wanted the baby to be born. When I arrived, I found Michal in labor on the ground level of the house, in the round TV room under the stairs, on a mattress, leaning on a beanbag, trying to find a comfortable position. The contractions were coming every three minutes and seemed strong and painful. Michal spent a lot of time in the toilet. When I examined her at 1:50 she was already four centimeters dilated and 100% effaced. She asked us to set up the pool.

Ohad got the pool, cleaned it and started blowing it up in the spacious upstairs bathroom. I was downstairs with Michal most of the time, massaging her back and breathing with her. Every once in a while, I would go up the spiral staircase to see what sort of progress Ohad was making with the pool and get my equipment set up. I had a feeling that things were moving quickly.

At 2:45 her waters broke spontaneously. Michal asked me to examine her, and after we heard the baby's heart tones, I checked her, even though I thought it could wait. She seemed too quiet and composed to have progressed significantly. But I was wrong. She was nine centimeters dilated; the head was at S+1. Ohad had just finished filling up the pool, and for a moment we didn't know whether or not Michal would even have enough time to enjoy using it.

She decided to make a mad dash up the stairs in between contractions, stripping off her clothes on the way up. She jumped into the pool, and at exactly 3 am the baby was born in the warm water. Everything was perfect.

The speed of the birth stunned us all. Michal had anticipated a long, difficult birth like her first. She had prepared me for hysterics and drama, but none of that happened. She had a simple, straightforward, wonderful physiological birth. Ohad was shocked by the speed of the events but delighted with the outcome. He had believed in Michal all along. She stayed in the pool together with the baby and enjoyed the warm water and the victory.

When she was ready, and after a nice shower, we moved Michal and baby Boaz over to the bed. Her identical twin sister arrived to take care of her, greet the baby and clean the house. They were alike and different as twins often are. It was as if Michal had an extension of herself. She was every woman's dream, another two hands, two feet and a body that wasn't pregnant or giving birth and could do whatever was necessary while Michal was busy falling in love with Boaz.

I felt very redundant very quickly, and after doing my minimal midwifery duties, I left Michal and Ohad and drove home. I still had some time to sleep before the sun would rise. Two births in six hours. Wow.

Lessons learned:
1. Second births can be REAL quick.
2. A small house? A big house? A crowded house? A new, beautifully designed house? What does it really matter? Love and support are the only things that make a difference; they enable the birthing woman to feel safe enough to open up and let the fruit of her womb drop off her tree.
3. Sometimes it is difficult to understand how quickly a woman is progressing by observing her behavior. If a woman asks to be examined, she probably has a reason, and that request should be honored.
4. Having a twin sister come to help in the house after a birth could be an idea for a start-up company. It doesn't get any better than that.

Backing Up and Backing Off

Sarahle phoned me one cold and rainy winter evening and asked me if I could cover for her because she was at a birth and clearly couldn't be in two places at the same time. I agreed to help her out even though the conditions were less than optimal.

No details concerning Liat's pregnancy were available to me except the fact that this was her first pregnancy, that she was 42+4 weeks and that she hadn't seen a doctor in four days. I was also told that her husband Yosi was less than happy about the birth taking place at home in their high-rise apartment in the French Carmel neighborhood of Haifa.

I was exhausted from teaching all day at the Midwifery course at Tel Hashomer, and I tried to see if Maya was available. She wasn't; she also had a woman in labor. It turned out that Lihi was also at a birth covering for Ronit, who was also at a birth. It was a busy night in the home birth world of northern Israel.

Avner had a bad feeling about this birth, but I had committed to going, and so I went. I got my equipment together and drove toward Haifa. I talked with Maya on the way, and she had considered coming with me but decided not to in the end. She wanted to be rested for the birth that she anticipated would start during the night. As I got to the portion of the trip that was unfamiliar to me, I called Yosi and had him direct me over the phone.

He waited for me on the sidewalk of their quiet street in a neighborhood filled with unusually tall apartment buildings. It was bitter cold, and the wind was coming up from the sea and howling through the buildings. It was dark, and the streets were empty. Yosi greeted me with the announcement that there was no electricity in the apartment but that he would try and fix it. Perhaps too many heaters were on at the same time. My thoughts jumped to the book *Midwives* in which a home birth midwife performs an emergency C-section in a log cabin in a snowstorm with no electricity or phone service. I had a sinking feeling in my gut.

Yosi helped me with my bags. He appeared to be in his late forties to mid-fifties. We entered the apartment. I dropped the bags and went to introduce myself to Liat. She understood that I was the midwife who would be taking over for Sarahle. The apartment was dark and cold. Liat was in a nightgown and a bathrobe. Her friend Alison and her sister Dafna were with her. I spotted Yosi's 16-year-old son in his bedroom with his head buried in a book.

Liat was having contractions every three minutes, and she was dealing with them on her hands and knees while being massaged by Dafna and Alison. Yosi solved the problem with the electricity but still seemed a little anxious. He kept himself busy by serving tea and cookies. Liat ushered me to the back room where she planned to give birth.

The room was small, dark and barely warmed by a small space heater. There was a thin mattress on the floor covered with a plastic tablecloth and a sheet. Liat showed me the under pads she had sewn for the birth, one layer of plastic table cloth and one layer of an old sheet sewn together by hand. It was obvious to me that she had put a lot of thought and effort into preparing for this birth.

I asked for some more light, and Yosi brought in a desk lamp which he put on the floor. Liat leaned on the railing of the baby's crib during the contractions. We heard the baby's heartbeat, even though it was difficult to find because of an anterior placenta. It sounded fine and was between 125-145 bpm. I examined her internally; her cervix was dilated one cm., and was 90% effaced. The last estimated fetal weight was four kilograms. She was disappointed about the lack of progress, and I was concerned about the baby's size in comparison with her height, which was 156 cm.

We joined the others in the living room. I saw that Liat was well supported by her sister and friend, so I asked for her documents and took the time to sit alone at the kitchen table and go through her pregnancy follow up. Everything seemed to be okay except for an isolated incident of high blood pressure at 37 weeks without any additional signs of preeclampsia. I took her blood pressure, and it was 140/90. After trying to help her to calm down, breathe and relax, I measured it again, and it was again 140/90. I could see on her face an expression of doom. She suspected that her home birth might be over, but neither of us said anything just yet.

Liat felt the urge to urinate, so I gave her a stick to test for proteinuria. She couldn't do it because there was only one bathroom in the apartment and Yosi's son was in there. She didn't feel comfortable knocking on the door and asking him to hurry up. He was in the shower, complaining that there was no hot water. Eventually, he came out, and Liat went in. She came out holding in her hand a stick showing protein ++. At this point, I felt myself approaching my red line. My negative intuitive feeling turned into a seemingly impossible situation: no heat, no electricity, no hot water and in the background the wind was still whistling ominously through the windows. There was no real labor progress; we had a disgruntled husband, an ornery teenage boy, high blood pressure and proteinuria.

I asked Liat to come into the back room with me for a talk, and she knew what I was about to say even before I opened my mouth. I broke the news as gently as I could, but she had to know that this birth could not continue at home. She was not surprised and was clearly more concerned about her own health and the baby's welfare than anything else. I quickly wrote a transfer letter and read it to her. Within ten minutes, they were all in the car on the way to the hospital. I could think of no reason for me to accompany them, so I went home.

When I got home, I called and spoke to Dafna. Liat was in the delivery room, and the staff was putting in an IV line and taking blood tests. I debated over and over in my head if I had transferred her for good reasons, or was it mostly because of the uneasy feeling in my gut. There was nothing more I could do, so I went to sleep.

I called Sarahle in the morning. Liat had been operated on at 1:20 am, and the baby was in the Neonatal Intensive Care Unit but was okay.

The presenting monitor showed clear signs of fetal distress, and they quickly decided on an emergency C-section. The baby's Apgar score was 5/9: not horrible but not good. I spoke with Liat, and she thanked me for saving her baby's life. I was confused, scared and relieved, a myriad of emotions, thoughts and sensations.

My reason for sending her to the hospital turned out to be unrelated to what panned out in the end. This is often the case in transfers; there is an explicit reason for the transfer, and as the birth unfolds the implicit reason presents itself. Most important was that the baby and mother were fine. The birth weight was 3.180 kilograms, not so big after all.

Lessons learned:

1. This birth was about intuition, fate, proper backup and protocols, like taking blood pressure at every birth immediately after hearing fetal heart sounds.
2. I am still trying to put my finger on exactly what felt wrong when I walked into that house. I know that the feeling in the pit of my stomach was impossible to misinterpret and that it ominously predicted distress.
3. I felt like we were all being sucked into a dangerous vortex and needed to find our way out. The high blood pressure showed up just in time and saved the life of that baby. Liat fulfilled her dream to become the mother of a healthy baby boy, and I was able to continue practicing midwifery for as long as I chose. I shudder to think of what might have happened if we had stayed at home, or if I hadn't taken her blood pressure.
4. Back-up is a sticky issue, and I think a lot about how to do it properly. I did not know this woman before I stepped foot in her apartment with the intention of delivering her baby.
5. Continuity of care and familiarity are two of the basic premises of the home birth advantage, and when an unknown back-up midwife is brought in, these advantages are lost.

> The players are the same, and the stage is the same, but the conductor of the orchestra is substituted at the last minute, and it changes the quality of the music.

I have had both good and bad experiences with backups. When I found myself in the impossible position of not being able to be in two places at the same time I, too, called in backup midwives to substitute for me. In over fifteen years, this didn't happen often, but when it did it was accompanied by weighty feelings of disappointment, guilt, frustration and anger. After months of working on creating a relationship, fate takes a turn and brings a stranger into the picture.

Some women know how to ease everyone's suffering by wielding a fatalistic approach, believing that it was meant to be and that God has a mysterious plan that is unknown to all of us. Other women feel abandoned and never get beyond the feeling of betrayal. It took years to stop taking responsibility for things I cannot control like the serendipitous nature of birthing women's hormones and the synchronicity of the universe.

Surprise!

Miri was in the 25th week of her third pregnancy when we first met. She had birthed at home two years before and had experienced a miscarriage between that birth and this pregnancy. She was healthy and seemed content with herself, her son Nimrod, her relationship with her husband Noam and with her life in general. She was home-schooling Nimrod and so far, seemed to have achieved inspiring results. Nimrod is a radiant, curious, capable and expressive child who is an absolute pleasure to be with.

Throughout the pregnancy, our meetings were short and to the point; there was no delving into deep emotional issues or traumas. Each time we parted, I was left with the feeling that she enjoyed our interaction, but that she didn't really need me. We breezed through the pregnancy with a minimal number of short meetings which were pleasant enough and sort of businesslike.

One issue that did pervade our discussions was who would be with her during the labor. Her parents had attended her first birth. She and Noam related the story as a positive experience but were hesitant to repeat it. Miri yearned for a more intimate experience and contemplated being alone with only her partner and me. Apparently, the first birth had been too much of a crowd scene. Up until the very end, I didn't know what her decision was.

When she was 39 weeks, I learned from a phone conversation with Miri that her father was going into the hospital for cardiac surgery, so she didn't have to tell her parents that she didn't want them at the birth after all. That problem solved itself. The next issue was what to do with Nimrod. That also remained unsolved until the last minute.

Saturday morning, I called Miri just to say hello and get a feeling for what was going on. She was feeling fine and was experiencing no hints of oncoming labor. Her father had undergone the surgery and was recovering. He was expected to return home on Sunday. That night, at about midnight, her contractions began.

Miri called me at about 5:45 am with contractions every five minutes. She explained that they were getting longer, but she was still unsure about whether or not it was time for me to come. I was up anyway, and she knew that today would be the day that she would give birth, so we decided that I would get ready and come over. Her request was that I do so slowly, that there was no need to rush.

I cooperated. I took my time getting out of bed, took a nice long shower, gave thought and effort to getting dressed slowly, made myself a cup of coffee and reread her documents. By the time I packed the car and left the house, it was 6:45, an hour since she had called. When I was on the road, I called to tell them that I was on my way. I spoke with Noam who was glad to hear that I was coming because the contractions were getting stronger.

At about 7:00 I approached the traffic light at Kfar Manda and saw smoke, fire, sprays of water and a fire truck blocking the intersection. As I got closer, I could see that an automobile was on fire and that there was no way I could get through the intersection because the police had blocked it off. I called Noam to tell him what was happening, while I turned around to go back to the Hamovil Intersection and head in the direction of Shfaram and Iblin. There was no other way to get to their house.

At about 7:15 I found myself in a seemingly endless stream of cars that were almost at a standstill approaching Shfaram. I called Noam again to tell him where I was, and this time I heard Miri roaring in the background. The contractions had become intense, and I broke out in a hot sweat as I understood what was happening and what would be the outcome. She would be having this baby without me. It was crystal clear. I had no real option other than to sit in this traffic jam which was barely even moving. It was Sunday morning rush hour at Somech Intersection, and I was in the middle of it.

We spoke again after another five minutes. The birth was becoming more and more imminent. Noam asked me what to do. I advised him to get Miri to put a finger in her vagina and report what she felt.

The answer came back immediately; it was something round, hard and slippery, the head. What to do now? Orders poured out of me. "Put a mattress on the floor, spread out the under pads, make sure that Miri is comfortable, have cotton diapers close by, prepare to catch the baby, don't let her fall, put the phone on speaker, you can do this."

I finally made my way through the intersection and was racing towards Ibilin. Noam was on speaker phone. I tried to calm him down, calm myself down, concentrate on giving him good instructions and drive without getting into an accident, all at the same time. As I approached Iblin, Miri could feel the head, and a minute later, the baby was born into her arms. Noam had gone to the bathroom to bring her a hot compress for her perineum and had missed the instant of the birth. I heard the baby's cry over the speakerphone in my car and breathed a brief sigh of relief. Everything sounded fine. It was a girl. The time was 7:40.

I arrived at their home at 7:50 and was greeted by Noam as he bounded out of the house to help me with my bags. I found Miri in the family room, radiant, holding the baby in her arms, sitting in a puddle of blood and amniotic fluid, looking very proud of herself. I got my wits about me quickly, cleaned up and helped her to get more comfortable. A few minutes later, I separated the cord and helped her get the placenta out. One dose of Arnica, and everything was fine. She had a small nick that didn't require suturing. Nimrod was still fast asleep in his bed and didn't even know that his new baby sister had arrived.

Miri got into the bathtub and cleaned herself off, took the baby in there with her and she immediately took the breast. Noam got the camera and took lots of pictures. It really was quite a sight.

After a few cups of tea and some apple cake, when we all settled into a calmer mode, Miri told me that this was the birth she had dreamed of, unassisted, not even by a midwife. She hadn't dared to tell the world beforehand and to actually plan it this way, but this was her fantasy birth. And she got it. A car on fire helped. Things have a way of working themselves out.

Lessons learned:
1. An important lesson I learned from this birth, which I will continue to learn over and over, is that we have no control over most of the things that happen in our lives. It is vital to trust that everything will work out for the best.
2. A baby that arrives so quickly and easily usually doesn't need any help from anyone.
3. It was no wonder that I felt unnecessary during the pregnancy. I turned out to be pretty unnecessary at the birth too.
4. It makes me very happy when a woman gets what she wishes for. I was happy for Miri that she got the birth she wanted, even though it was at the expense of my blood pressure and coronary arteries.

Giving Birth in Peace

Orit and Israel first approached me after I returned from the States for my nephew's wedding. Orit wanted to give birth at home, but Israel had some fears concerning the issue. In addition, Orit's mother is a certified nurse-midwife, and a decision to give birth at home would entail the price of dealing with her criticism. But as we talked, I could feel that Israel's fears were negotiable and that, as a couple, they were leaning in the direction of home birth.

In the meantime, the second Lebanese war broke out. Seventeen members of Avner's family moved in with us to distance themselves from the missiles showering their homes near the Lebanese border. We were inundated; there were people everywhere. My dining room table looked like Thanksgiving for three weeks. My refrigerator was overrun with food and produce that the women had grabbed minutes before leaving their homes. It was overwhelming, and it wasn't just because of the crowded quarters. Tempers were short with so much fear and anxiety in the air.

I traveled to Beer Sheva for five days to begin my training in Somatic Experiencing. During a lunch break, I received a phone call from Israel and Orit. They had decided that they wanted to plan a home birth with me. Orit had a few health issues, none of which was serious enough to prevent her from birthing at home, but they each required some attention. She had a thyroid problem, her platelet count was low and getting lower and her blood pressure was a little high, around 135/85.

Orit is a yoga teacher; she is highly aware of her body, very intelligent, well-read and well prepared for the birth, including having studied self-hypnosis. She was taking herbal medicines and getting acupuncture treatments for her thrombocytopenia. Her Ob/Gyn was closely following her case, and I consulted with him concerning her intention to give birth at home. He saw no reason why she couldn't plan a home birth.

After I returned from Beer Sheva, Orit, Israel and I met in one of the guest cabins in our backyard. My house was still overrun with Avner's family, and there were no quiet, private corners, so I opened up a clinic in one of the cabins. We had a good, long meeting there. In her complete blood count there were some abnormal values; both her hemoglobin and mean – platelet volume were high. This could be a sign of developing toxemia. The last thing I did before they went home was take her blood pressure again. It was 150/100, but with no protein in her urine. I explained the meaning of this and asked them to measure it again in the morning and let me know.

Orit had no support people in mind other than Israel, and I asked them if they might be interested in having a midwifery student join us for the birth. They agree to consider it. The next morning her blood pressure was down to 120/75. We agreed to continue monitoring her blood pressure, do some more blood tests and try and see whether or not she was slowly developing toxemia. Our agreement was that if her platelets went below 100,000, she would go to the hospital for the birth. They investigated the possibility of Laniado Hospital in Netanya which had a good reputation for supporting natural birth.

The war raged on. Most of our contact was over the phone. I spoke with her doctor who I managed to reach in between his reserve duties. Orit and Israel left Haifa and went to Israel's parents' house in the South but soon returned home, with a positive attitude and an internal feeling of safety. She had blood tests done weekly. Her Hb and MPV were going up and her platelets were going down. In addition, total protein was going down and alkaline phosphatase was going up. After consulting Anne Frye's book *Understanding Diagnostic Tests in the Childbearing Year*, I understood that she might have a developing case of toxemia, but it still wasn't explicit enough to warrant hospital care. Her blood pressure was stable and she felt good. Our fingers were crossed that things wouldn't get worse, but my feeling was that they might. In addition, they informed me that they had decided that they were interested in having the midwifery student, Anat, join us at the birth and asked me for her phone number.

Orit entered her 39th week, and we all decided that it was time to meet: Orit, Israel, Anat and I. It had been quiet for ten days in Haifa with no Katusha rockets and no medium-range missiles. We set up a meeting for 8 pm at Orit and Israel's house. As the time approached, my stomach got tight with anxiety. It's hard for me to say whether it was intuition, fear or instinct, but I received a very clear message from my body not to go to that meeting.

After a week in Beer Sheva at the SE training, I had become acutely aware of my body sensations, and my body was saying, "No". Israel tried to calm my fears and told me that everything was okay, that outside children were playing and riding bicycles, and that I should come and that I should feel safe. I asked him if his optimism was for sale. His response was, "Don't be so quick to buy. Maybe you're right, and I'm the fool."

I deliberated over this for a while, and at about 7 pm, I decided not to go. A few minutes later, the sirens went off, one after the next, and things got crazy. While I was on the phone with Anat, she went into her family's safe room in Haifa. I talked with Orit while she was in a bomb shelter. At about 7:50 pm a missile fell in Hadar, near Bnai Zion Hospital, that set off a huge fire. Missiles fell in Carmel Center, Nesher and who knows where else. I would have been on the road in the car if I hadn't listened to my body.

A few days later, Avner's family decided to take a trip to Jerusalem for the weekend, all 17 of them. The exodus took place mid-morning, and for an hour or two, I went from room to room, making sure they hadn't left anyone behind.

That evening Avner went to synagogue, and while he was praying for peace and the safety of our community and country, several missiles fell in the fields of our moshav. The boom shook the windows of my house; it was almost like an earthquake. I jumped like a terrified rabbit into our safe room downstairs and waited for Avner to come home.

He helped me to calm myself, and after I managed to do so, we both realized how hungry we were. We decided to celebrate both being alive and his family's departure by going out to eat. During dinner, the sirens went off again, and we were ushered into the meat freezer, which was determined to be the safest part of the restaurant. Could things get any crazier?

Exactly one week later, on August 14, a ceasefire went into effect. I sat on my back porch listening to the luxurious silence of the absence of sirens, helicopters and airplanes. I called Orit to set a date to meet that evening. She read me the results of yesterday's blood tests; her platelets were going down, now 86,000. The result wasn't critical, but I still had a sinking feeling in my chest. I was worried about Orit's health and the baby's well-being. I felt that something wasn't right.

All day long, I ruminated over her test results, my fears, my issues concerning boundaries and my ability to be true to myself. I didn't think that it was safe for her to have the baby at home. I felt that she would be better off in the hospital. I went to meet her in order to tell her that. I knew it wouldn't be easy for any of us to have this discussion.

It was my first time in their apartment. There was a lot of wood, an interesting blend of Indian art and antique furniture. We walked through the apartment and discussed where to locate the birthing pool and how to move the furniture in order to make more room. I felt like an imposter, participating in this discussion when I knew that I had to initiate a much more crucial conversation that would preempt all others. We settled down in the living room with Israel's great coffee, and when they finished asking questions, I took over.

I told them that I was nervous about Orit having the baby at home, that her blood tests were getting more pathological and that as the birth approaches, they most probably will get worse and not better. I explained the implications of preeclampsia again, trying not to scare them and hoping they would understand.

They remained firm in their optimism and tried to bring me over to their side. I recalled the evening a week before when I almost bought Israel's optimism and then decided to act on my own instincts instead. I understood that I had to be very clear, and very assertive. I had no other choice, and neither did they.

After accepting the circumstances of the new reality, the discussion moved on to choosing a hospital and what care Orit should expect to receive there. As we talked, we all noticed that she was having contractions, at first every five minutes and then very quickly developing into every three minutes. In between contractions I took her blood pressure. It was high, 170/110 but with no signs of toxemia, protein in her urine, headaches, stomach aches, dizziness or vision problems. She felt fine, and her contractions were getting more intense by the minute.

I phoned Anat to find out what the situation was like at L&D at Carmel Hospital. Both the delivery rooms at Carmel and at Rambam were still underground because of the war. Orit vetoed both of them.

I called Bnai Zion Hospital. It was about 10:30 pm, and the staff was about to switch from evening to night shift and the delivery room was empty. We started to get organized for our move over to the hospital. In the meantime, Orit was nauseous and threw up a few times. I had a feeling she was progressing really quickly.

I performed an internal exam and found her cervix four centimeters dilated, 100% effaced. Only half an hour had passed since the first contraction. I made it clear to them that we needed to get this wagon train moving. We took my car. Israel drove.

We entered the delivery room as the midwives from the evening shift left to go home. Ragda and Tal were our options. Both were absolutely fine with me, and at first, it seemed that Ragda would be with us. Orit said that she needed the toilet, and Ragda took her to the bathroom of the natural delivery suite. I came in afterward, and we quickly found ourselves alone there.

A few minutes later, Tal came in and left, and again we were alone. This was actually exactly what Orit wanted all along, to be left alone. She was on the toilet for a while and then found a comfortable position on her hands and knees on the floor of the bathroom. She wasn't budging, and she was beginning to feel pressure.

Her waters broke spontaneously all over the floor of the bathroom. There was meconium in the amniotic fluid, which is not a good sign. I went to look for Tal. It was time to become more vocal and more assertive. We had come to the hospital for medical supervision. Since we had arrived, there had been no such supervision, just a birthing woman laboring on the floor of the bathroom.

What was the advantage of being in the hospital if this was the case? My memory jumped to a memory of the wise Dr. Levinsky telling stories about women having eclamptic fits on the toilet.

I asked Tal to come in; I told her about the meconium and asked her to help me to move Orit into a room, onto a bed and hooked up to a fetal monitor. Tal is a very tall woman. With her hands on her hips, she loudly and assertively declared the need for Orit to be in a room, on the bed and hooked up to the monitor. Orit obeyed.

We could hardly get a heartbeat. The head was very low down, and we were hearing end-stage bradycardia, possibly a sign of fetal distress. Tal examined Orit and affirmed it: nine cm. dilated, 100% effaced, the head S+1. I was relieved to know that she would be giving birth soon.

We were all excited, but everyone else was panicking. The junior resident came into the room and started threatening to initiate a C-section. He wasn't informed about the nine cm. The senior resident came in and said that he wanted the baby out now. All of a sudden and all at once, an IV line was put in, blood tests were taken, blood pressure measured, and admitting forms were filled.

Orit was deep in outer (or inner) space and couldn't relate to any of this pandemonium. She was feeling pressure and started pushing. Israel was gone; he had been sent downstairs to get stickers. I was with Orit trying to keep her centered and pushing, while the staff did their job and dealt with the bureaucracy. The senior physician wanted to do a vacuum delivery, and I wanted to get that baby out before he succeeded. In the meantime, the midwife shaved her in preparation for an episiotomy and a vacuum delivery.

The urge to push became overwhelming, and Orit started pushing like crazy. Israel returned with the stickers. The heartbeat was consistently low, and the doctor was dressed and getting ready to do the vacuum. In the meantime, Orit pushed the baby down to the perineum, an episiotomy was cut without notification or permission and the baby girl popped right out, with her cord around her neck but just fine. Her Apgar score was 9/10. Orit was ecstatic, Israel was in shock and everyone else was relieved that everything was okay. Noam was born at 11:45 pm, less than an hour from the time we arrived in the delivery room, less than four hours from the first contraction.

Suddenly, the irony of the whole situation hit me. I couldn't help but wonder if Orit had been desperately holding onto her pregnancy so that she could give birth to her baby in a time of peace. Or maybe Noam finally felt that it was safe to come out.

Thankfully, Orit's blood pressure stabilized after the birth, and she never developed toxemia.

Lessons learned:
1. Listening to my intuition paid off again. It is important to listen to the whispers and not wait for the shouts.
2. Just like in Limor's birth, it was surprising to witness Orit going into labor, especially because there wasn't the slightest hint beforehand. This reinforces my understanding of how the cognitive, emotional and physical elements of our existence are intertwined.
3. Tensions created by the threat of war affect each and every citizen of the country being threatened, including the pregnant women and the babies in their wombs. It was not a coincidence that Orit went into labor one day after the ceasefire.
4. Even though I am gaining experience as a home birth midwife, it is still difficult for me to be the one to declare the need to move over to the hospital. It is never easy to be the one to destroy a woman's dream of a home birth, even though I know it is in her best interest. I still need to do a lot of work on the issue of boundaries.

Not Here to Make Friends

It took a long time before I found the courage to write down the chain of events of Ela's birth. While on vacation in Florida, after participating in a *Mayan Abdominal Massage* workshop, I found the motivation and courage to document the story of this birth, my scariest birth ever.

The host of the workshop was a relatively young home birth midwife. During one of the lunch breaks, we were exchanging birth stories, and she shared some words of wisdom that fell on my attentive ears. Recently she had transferred a woman to the hospital and was treated poorly by the emergency medical service people. She reacted by continuing to be assertive and communicative, even though she felt that they had been rude. Then she told me exactly what she said to them, "I'm not here to make friends. I'm here to get this baby out." It was so simple and so wise, and it echoed over and over again in my mind.

The next day, I asked her if that bit of wisdom was her own. The answer was, "No." These words had been passed on to her at the beginning of her midwifery training by one of her clinical instructors. It helped her to maintain a safe emotional distance from her clients so that she could do her job well. I needed to hear this and felt that I needed to learn how to do this better. I sometimes find myself too emotionally involved with my clients, and I do not serve them as well as I should because I am busy getting close to them.

At the time, I was also reading *Listen to Me Good: The Life Story of an Alabama Midwife*, and something struck me in the book. The narrator is adamant that she doesn't want to become a midwife, even though she has been practicing midwifery for a long, long time. She is then told by an older midwife that she is doing this work because the Lord wants her to, and if it wasn't right for her, she wouldn't have the knowledge or stamina for it.

That also struck a tone somewhere deep inside me. If this wasn't right for me, I wouldn't be doing it. I wouldn't be able to do whatever was necessary to move forward: learning, teaching, and gaining more and more knowledge each and every day. It wouldn't pull at me in the way it does. It wouldn't obsess my mind the way it does. It wouldn't be the one thing that interests me more than anything else on Earth. Being a midwife is a lot of responsibility and is sometimes very scary. Ela's birth was terrifying and traumatic for everyone involved, but we all tried to learn our lessons and move forward.

When I first met Ela, I saw a bold, honest, creative and beautiful young woman who was highly motivated to give birth at home. She was 24 years old, and at the time her relationship with her partner Max was unstable. He wasn't sure whether he wanted to be in a committed relationship and wasn't sure that he was ready to become a father. During the pregnancy, they had many disagreements on these topics, and Ela eventually moved out of their house and into a small living unit in her parents' backyard. Her family supported her unconditionally. Up until the final moment, none of us knew whether or not Max would be at the birth. Because of this uncertainty, I felt the need to create a strong connection with Ela so that in the case of Max's possible absence, I would be there to provide her with the emotional support that every birthing woman deserves. A single mom who knew that she would be alone could prepare herself and ask her girlfriends to be with her at her birth. This was not the case, and the ambiguity made it difficult to plan.

For me the birth began with a phone call from Max; Ela was having contractions. They weren't sure that they needed my presence yet, but it sounded like things were beginning to gain momentum. I was at home in bed sleeping. It was early Saturday morning, the night between the third and fourth day of a long, drawn-out induction at Nazareth Hospital. I didn't know how I was going to manage both a home birth in a village near Carmiel and a hospital birth in Nazareth. I got ready to go along for the ride to see how things would unfold. I felt a mild sensation of trepidation in my chest and tried to calm myself by saying over and over that everything will work itself out.

When I arrived, Ela was in her little house in the backyard of her parents' home. She was having contractions every five minutes, and they seemed painful. She was having difficulty communicating verbally both with me and with Max, but she somehow managed to express that she wanted to move over to the big house and find a new spot.

I examined her and found that she was four centimeters dilated. We were all happy with her progress and slowly migrated over to the big house. We brought the pool upstairs and blew it up. In the meantime, Ela got into the shower and began to find her rhythm in the new venue.

Ela and Max were good together, so I left them alone, went downstairs and had breakfast with her parents. They were excited and a little anxious but were doing okay. This was all new for them, and they were highly motivated to support their daughter in any and every way necessary. They were thrilled about becoming grandparents.

Ela entered the pool and enjoyed the feel of the water and Max's presence. She progressed nicely and eventually left the pool to walk around. She responded intuitively to the needs of her body in a simple and uncomplicated manner.

I was exhausted and not completely present after spending parts of three days at the hospital with Dana. As the morning progressed into noon, Dana was still at the hospital, and my thoughts were with her. I wondered if I would be there to support her through another day of induction attempts. I hesitated to tell each of the women about the other. I ended up telling Dana about Ela because I had no choice. I did not tell Ela about Dana, though she might have sensed something. I was distracted and spent a lot of time on the phone, sending and receiving text messages, trying to cover all bases. Dana assured me that she was okay, that she felt comfortable with the midwifery staff at the hospital, and was well supported by her partner and her sister. I still felt torn.

Three of the four private Nazareth midwives were sleeping after night shifts. The fourth was working a morning shift at the hospital. No one was available to back me up with Dana. Lihi was the only one who agreed to join me as the second midwife with Ela, but only on the condition that she could bring her baby. She told me that she was at home, relaxing with her family and was waiting for my call. I called her when Ela was nine centimeters dilated at about noon.

It turned out to be a long time before the baby was born. He was bigger than anyone had estimated, and it took about two and a half hours for Ela to push him out. She was exhausted; she lost and regained her patience several times along the way. I had learned through our prenatal visits that she was good at short, intensive efforts but was less proficient with long, continuous ones. In this predicament, she had no choice, and she understood that she had to do this, even though she didn't like it and was exhausted.

The sun was beating through the bedroom window. In the yard, Ela's parents, brother and sister sat together with Lihi and her baby and heard Ela grunting and pushing her baby out. They were chatting and passing the time, while Ela was making the effort of her lifetime. Max was very supportive. The contractions were coming relatively far apart, at six-minute intervals.

The head was on the perineum for over a half-hour. I also lost and regained my patience several times. In the back of my mind, I was also thinking of Dana and how I planned to go to Nazareth after this birth was over. I felt my presence drifting in and out as I sat on the bed in the sunlight and waited for this big baby boy to break through into the world.

Eventually, it happened. Ela got very serious about pushing and made it happen. He arrived in all his glory. The umbilical cord was tight around his neck, but Ela kept pushing, and I unwound the cord after the baby was out. He cried and was good and healthy and big. He weighed almost four kilograms.

Max was in awe of Ela. Ela was blown away by the enormity and intensity of the experience, and she was exhausted. She had used every bit of energy in her being to give birth. She took the baby into her arms and held him to her breast. She tried to regain her center.

We waited for the placenta. After about fifteen minutes, she told us that she felt pressure and the need to push. The placenta was delivered inside out. The sac was intact and filled with blood, maybe 750 ml, maybe even more. It spilled onto the under pad and beyond, staining the bedsheets.

I massaged Ela's uterus, and she continued to bleed. The blood was bright red. Her uterus felt well contracted, but she kept on bleeding. Max saw the amount of blood and was terrified. Time stood still for a moment. I called out to Lihi from the window and told her to come quickly. She left her baby downstairs with Ela's family and came upstairs. I went back to massaging her uterus again, and blood was still gushing out. It was bright red, almost orange and was pouring out of her. I was scared. So was Lihi. I had never had a hemorrhage at a home birth where I was the primary midwife, and I had never seen blood this color. This situation caught me completely off guard.

We started by trying to insert an IV line; this turned out to be a mistake. Lihi put the first line in, which wasn't well placed, and pulled it out. The second attempt wasn't in the vein either and was also pulled out. The third attempt worked, and we added Pitocin to contract the uterus and stop the bleeding. When I stood up, I stepped into a cold puddle of IV fluids that had dripped onto the floor. I felt the panic spread through my body like an electric shock, from my wet foot straight up to my heart. This was not a good situation. We needed to act now!

It is almost impossible to recount the events in their proper order because my mind doesn't remember them in that way. This is what happens after a traumatic event. Everything is a blur, a chaotic mosaic of memories. My written notes helped me to piece together the details of the event afterward.

We called the ambulance service. Lihi took that initiative, and it was blessed and critical. I gave Ela an intramuscular shot of Pitocin in her leg with a needle that was too big. She got the Methergine shot in her second leg with the right-sized needle. Her blood pressure was below mentioning.

The bleeding turned into clotting. She got a few doses of homeopathic Arnica. We put an oxygen mask over her face. She was on the verge of fainting but through a superhuman effort somehow managed to stay conscious and focused. We held her legs high to send more blood to her head and heart. She never lost consciousness, and this was encouraging. Her sister took the baby. Her family was terribly frightened as were we all.

For a brief moment, I missed the delivery room. I missed the team and the availability of immediate help in emergency situations. I missed being able to call out in distress and having the luxury of too many people barging into the room in response to my call for help. I missed sharing the responsibility and the need for action with trained medical doctors.

The ambulance arrived. They found fault in some of the things we had done. The oxygen flow rate wasn't strong enough (should have been 10 liters/min, not 5 liters/min). They wanted to replace the Pitocin drip with a clean bag with no drugs. We argued with them not to change the bag, contending that the contractions of the uterus that the Pitocin provided were essential. The oxygen tank should have been lying down so that it wouldn't fall. They were right about that.

Ela's blood pressure and pulse slowly improved. I found a few moments to examine the placenta. It was big and with no apparent missing pieces. We gathered the placenta into a plastic bag so we could take it with us to the hospital. I called the delivery room to tell them that we were on the way. While on the phone, I looked out the window and saw Lihi's baby alone in the sun in the yard, apparently asleep.

The ambulance crew seemed a bit phlegmatic and were rather annoying. They asked Ela twice to stand up and climb onto the trolley. I know they would have managed if she had been unconscious and needed to be carried, so why weren't they helping her? Finally, we were in the ambulance and moving in the direction of the hospital. I said a little prayer for Ela.

We were well received in the delivery room. The doctors were kind and efficient. We were not praised for anything we had done, but they noticed that we had brought her in quickly and in stable condition. The midwives were wonderful and very supportive. I was happy and relieved to be in the hospital.

The hunch was that there was a cervical tear. The decision was made to do both a manual revision of the uterus and the cervix. This involved checking the inner wall of the uterus for retained pieces of the placenta and checking the cervix for an injured, bleeding artery. Nothing was found. Eventually, with enough Pitocin, the bleeding stopped. The official diagnosis was uterine atony, which seemed so mundane considering how extraordinary this bleed had been.

Everywhere I turned I saw fear, anger, shock and trauma. It was an awful experience for Ela, Max, her parents, her siblings, Lihi and for me and my reflection in the mirror. Most of the time, I was so terrified that I couldn't even connect with myself. In between, I also felt some relief, because I knew that Ela was okay and clearly alive.

Ela received two pints of blood two days later. She felt like shit, had problems breastfeeding and was yellowish, weak and scared to death. The birth of the baby had been long and difficult but great; the aftermath was catastrophic and terrifying. I went to visit her twice, once on the day she came home from the hospital and again a few days later.

During the first visit, she was quiet, polite and focused on the breastfeeding challenge. She seemed a bit disconnected from the baby. During the second visit Ela's feelings poured out after she allowed herself to cry. She was devastated by the whole experience and had lots to say to me on a personal level. I will sum it up by saying that she was profoundly disappointed by how we handled the situation and by our panic. This strummed on a very deep heartstring because I, too, was profoundly disappointed by my own functioning.

This discussion with Ela sent me home devastated, and as a result, I entered a whirlwind of learning, reading and questioning, trying to understand what we did wrong, what we did right and how we could do it better the next time. I clearly understood that I had to do everything in my power in order not to panic in this manner ever again.

Postpartum hemorrhage (PPH) became my obsession and later my expertise. I ordered and read books. I met with a paramedic from the ambulance service and discussed the case. I met with Lihi, and together we rehashed the event, shared our thoughts and reactions and learned as much as we could. I read everything possible on the topic of uterine atony and PPH. I reacquainted myself with the pharmacology of Pitocin and Methergine. I talked with experienced homebirth midwives about their experiences with bleeds. I left no stone unturned on the topic.

My continued training in Somatic Experiencing provided me with tools to identify this as a potentially traumatizing event, recognize the signs and symptoms of post-trauma and promote healing in myself and in others. One of my greatest regrets is that I wasn't skilled enough at the time to help Ela work through the trauma of her birth experience. I didn't understand how much she needed my continued support following this very traumatic birth. I knew that she was angry and disappointed, and it was difficult for me to face her.

Ela's birth was clearly one of the most terrifying experiences in my career as a midwife. It rattled me to my core, and because of the manner in which I dealt with it, the end-product was more knowledge, more safety, more attention and more humility. It made me a better midwife.

A few years later Ela had her second baby at the hospital and bled again. In between births, she had minor surgery on her cervix and also bled. She never discovered the source of her propensity for bleeding despite numerous tests. Apparently, she has some sort of undiagnosed clotting disorder. She and Max remained a couple and created a family together.

Lessons learned:
1. When there is a long second stage and a big baby, it makes sense to expect that a bleed may happen. Have the drugs out and ready to give if necessary.

2. Pathology in birth exists. It is rare, but it happens. It took me too long to understand how serious this bleed was. It was totally unexpected.
3. There should be a clear division of labor when there is a bleed. The primary midwife massages the uterus constantly while communicating with the woman, explaining to her what is happening and calming her down. The second midwife, who is less emotionally involved, administers the drugs and inserts the IV lines.
4. Go straight for the uterus and don't stop massaging it until the bleeding stops. Massage from all directions, not just the fundus and give special attention to the sides, which is often the area where the placental insertion is.
5. While doing this, talk with the woman and make sure she understands what is happening and ask her to stop bleeding. It sounds like a strange request, but sometimes it works.
6. Within two minutes intramuscular Pitocin starts working. It is worthwhile to start with IM and then go on to insert the IV line afterward, knowing that the medicine is already working.
7. Giving oxygen takes very little time. The tank should be horizontal, and the flow should be open to 10 l/min until the reservoir fills up, then go down to 5 l/min. What is already lying down cannot fall.
8. When a bleeding woman is fainting, taking her blood pressure is a waste of precious time. It is going to be low, and you are already doing everything you can to raise it. Legs should be raised to help supply the brain and heart with blood.
9. Emotional over-attachment to clients puts everyone in jeopardy of less-than-optimal functioning in emergency situations. I think that I would have panicked less if I had been more emotionally distanced from Ela. This is still a tricky subject because I tend to become highly connected to my clients.

A Breath of Fresh Air

Ronit was referred to me by Chen, a delightful woman from Haifa who gave birth with me at home a few months earlier. When I first met Ronit, I could sense some of their similar qualities, a kind of energy that good girlfriends sometimes acquire from one another.

We met at her home because she had an 11-month-old baby and no transportation. Her house was cluttered and a bit chaotic, but she and her baby Raz were charming. I fell in love with both of them immediately. By the time I left their apartment in Carmel Center across the street from the auditorium, I felt that I had made two new friends.

The pregnancy was more or less eventless except that Raz got sick and was hospitalized. Breastfeeding women all over the North generously contributed their breast milk. Everything else was fine.

Ronit shared with me a list of positive affirmations that she had created in order to train her mind for a good birth. They were pasted on the doors of the bathroom, the refrigerator and the closet, all in plain view. The idea was to flood her mind with optimistic, healthy and positive thoughts, following the principles of Hypnobirthing, a birth preparation technique that had recently arrived in Israel. The skeptic in me smirked inwardly as I read the list. It sounded too good to be true.

- I give birth in the light.
- I give birth in love.
- I am surrounded by light.
- I breathe light.
- My body is calm, relaxed and ready to receive my baby.
- With each contraction, my body makes more room for my baby.
- I am confident.
- Each contraction is like a wave coming in and going out. I ride the waves.
- Each contraction brings me closer to my baby.
- My birth empowers me.

- I sing my baby out.
- I breathe my baby out.
- I relinquish control and let my body lead.

Ronit's birth came after I had accompanied several women in a few difficult and complicated labors, culminating in three transfers and a C-section. I needed a breath of fresh air and hoped Ronit's birth would provide it. Thursday morning we talked on the phone. She was 40+5 weeks. I half-jokingly asked her if a threat might help her to get motivated because on Sunday she would need to go to the hospital to do an ultrasound and monitor just to make sure everything is OK. She wasn't happy about the idea.

Friday morning, I woke up at 6:30 with a text message from Ronit: having contractions every 10 minutes. The threat worked. The next text was at 7:20: contractions every 5 minutes, getting stronger, Raz and Dotan are still asleep. Another one at 8:30: contractions every 3 minutes. It was time to get organized and moving.

I arrived at 9:20. Dotan had taken Raz to her grandparents' house. Ronit was alone, listening to music, laughing and smiling, happy as can be, organizing the house, getting ready for the birth, dancing and singing. She showed me photos she had taken of Raz at the beach the day before. She is totally in love with Raz who is her primary source of inspiration for the developing labor.

We flow from room to room, relocating piles of folded laundry, making room for my bags and clearing a space for the pool in the bedroom. Dotan calls every few minutes, once from the grandparents, twice from the supermarket, and once from the parking lot. The contractions are getting stronger, and Ronit wants him HOME. At about 10:00 he arrives and gets very busy following orders. He had no idea how quickly the birth was moving. This seems to be a very common occurrence in second births.

In the meantime, Ronit is dancing in her underpants to loud pop music playing full blast, smiling away and howling during contractions.

I managed to film a few minutes of this, and the short clip entitled "Dancing Through Labor" eventually went viral on YouTube and has over 30,000 views. At this point, I am getting ready for the birth because it seems to me that this baby is plowing its way out, even though I have not even examined her mom. I call Maya and tell her to get on the road; I have a strong feeling that we will not actually meet today.

The pool is ready at about 10:30. Ronit gets in the water which seems to be filling up very slowly. The water helps a bit, but the contractions are very strong and close together. Ronit feels her bones moving. She feels her back open. She feels the need to poop. She examines herself and feels the head very close. I examine her and find nine centimeters, 100% effaced, head at S+1. Her cervix is like butter.

She is on her knees when her waters break spontaneously, and immediately thereafter she feels the need to push. In this position, the water isn't deep enough for the head to be entirely submerged. She needs to flip over, and I ask her to do so. Her response is, "I can't move," but she has to. I help her to get into a squat, and the baby's head just slips onto her perineum. I gently open one knee to allow her to sit back and let the head slide all the way out. After a few seconds, the head turns, and the body is out. Ronit reaches out with both hands and catches her own baby. 10:56 is the time. We are all so excited that we forget to check to see if it is a girl or a boy. It's a girl, and she looks just like Raz.

Maya is somewhere in Carmel Center driving around and looking for a parking spot. We never did meet that morning because the placenta came out with no problem, and Maya turned around and drove home.

What a birth! It was an exhilarating experience of health, happiness, good energy and spirit. Ronit showered and got settled in bed. The baby immediately took the same breast that Raz had sucked on a few hours before. Dotan was in shock. He couldn't believe the speed of what had just happened. If the line at the supermarket had been just a little bit longer, he probably would have missed the birth.

I took Ronit's list of affirmations off the closet door and read it to myself and then again out loud. I couldn't wipe the smile off my face. Everything on the list had manifested itself. I had really needed this. I needed the affirmation of the ease with which babies CAN come into the world. It really was a breath of fresh air.

Musings after Ronit's birth:

I ask myself questions about this "ease." Who are these women who birth this way? Is it their minds? Their bodies? Their hormones? Their nervous systems? Their upbringing? Can this be taught? Is this acquired? Learned? Inherited? Throughout the years, I continued to ask these questions. Sometimes I can predict who will have a quick and easy "butter birth." Sometimes I am so off the mark that it is embarrassing. Every time I am wrong, I learn something new and smile to myself as I notice that the Universe continues to provide me with lessons to learn.

132 | Birth Days

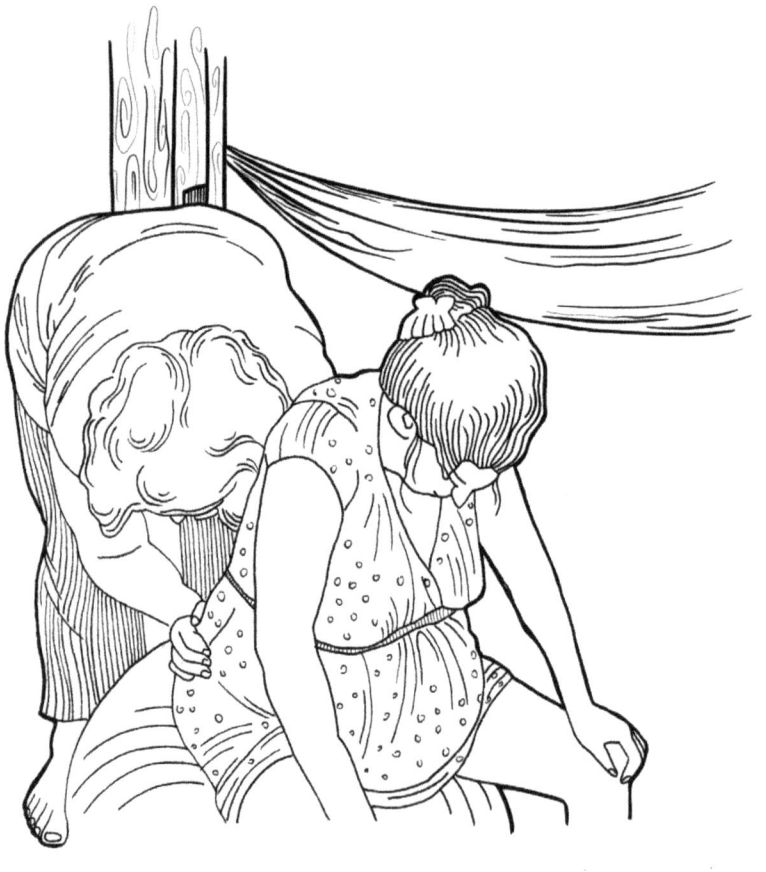

Births at Agoola

From the moment I heard the words "Birth Center" I knew that I wanted to be a part of one. The idea of working as a member of a team of like-minded midwives was very attractive. I visited birth centers in England, Germany, Jamaica and America and met with the midwives who were running them. I loved the energy, the soft, feminine atmosphere, the cooperation and the sense of community. These women had created centers where women before, during and after their births could find support, make new friends, feel at home and be a part of something bigger than themselves.

I was not alone. Other midwives in Israel were having similar thoughts and aspirations. Many attempts were made to secure permission from the Department of Health to create such birth centers but to no avail. The answer was always "No." Eventually, we went to the Knesset, the Israeli Parliament.

Journal Entry, July 7, 2004

Today was a big day. Midwives in flowered skirts graced the halls of the Israeli Knesset. We were there in order to sound our voices in the struggle to establish independent birth centers.

I don't think there has ever been a representation of midwives in the Knesset. They are usually too busy caring for women of various races and religions during their most challenging life event, their births. They are there in times of joy, pain, fear and sometimes even in times of crisis, war and natural disaster. They have had no free time to go to the Knesset to talk about their work, make a statement about their needs or even ask for anything. So, what has changed?

During the last twenty years, numerous midwives have submitted requests to open and establish birth centers. They visited such centers in other countries. They saw centers that meet the needs of healthy women who want to give birth in a homey atmosphere under the care of professional midwives without unnecessary interventions. Throughout the years these requests have been rejected by the Ministry of Health, stubbornly wielding its official policy against the establishment of birth centers.

Today we were there both for the women and for ourselves. We have licenses to work independently with pregnant women, but we have nowhere to do so. We want to get to know the women before we deliver their babies. We believe that birth can be a better and less traumatic experience if the birthing woman has the opportunity to receive continuous care by her midwife throughout her pregnancy and birth.

I firmly believe that Knesset members have been elected to serve the public and to make life better for the citizens they represent. I do not understand how endless refusals to establish birth centers serve the public. My understanding is that this policy serves only the hospitals which view birth as a business and refuse to share their power and money. Again, as usual, the women are the victims, both the mothers and the midwives.

There was a time when people died at home surrounded by their family and friends. Over time, death moved to hospitals. People began to end their lives among strangers attached to useless devices with no function other than to enable their caregivers to feel that something was being done. The fortunate ones died suddenly and at home without all this torture. Over time people consciously decided to die at home, and as a result, hospices were created. Today hospice care is considered the humane and preferable option.

At the beginning of life, the same principle is applicable. Some women are not fit to give birth in a hospital. Some of them choose to give birth at home with a midwife. Some give birth alone and unassisted because they can't afford to pay for a private midwife. Most will give birth in a hospital. Many of them will emerge with lingering negative reactions to their experiences. This will negatively affect their mothering, their relationships with their partners, their families and the communities they live in.

The future of our society is dependent upon the mental health of our mothers. Part of that health is grounded on the freedom of our mothers to make choices for their children according to their conscience, knowledge and intuition. Choosing how and where to give birth is a basic right. No one should be forced to give birth in a place that is not of their choice.

Today we went to the Knesset to talk about freedom of choice in birth. We did not invent this wheel. All over the world birth centers have been proven to be a safe, efficient and economical option. What are we waiting for? The time is ripe. The midwives are ready; the Department of Health isn't quite yet.

The Vision and the Construction

I decided not to wait for permission from the Department of Health. I dreamt about the building day and night. I gathered ideas and formulated a concept long before we even broke ground. In the end, the plan was mine. My architect thought it was a little off-the-wall, but he helped me transform my idea into a physical form. The design elements, inside and out, were inspired by the elements of earth, water and air. Construction took almost two years.

The living room is spacious and round. The kitchen is open and airy. The floor is made of sand-colored stone. There are many windows and doors allowing the light and wind to come through freely. The ceiling is high, and the lighting fixtures are porcelain. They create a pale, yellow light when they are lit.

The bedroom and the clinic are separated from the public space with double doors and a corridor. Inside, there is more intimacy. The rooms are closed off and private, the ceilings are lower and the windows are smaller. There is a huge, deep, custom-made bathtub in the bathroom off the bedroom with room enough for two. It is like a spring inside a cave.

The smallest details received as much attention as the larger ones: the paint color, the custom-made wooden furniture, a floor-to-ceiling hand-painted wall mural of a big blue wave, lots of pillows of various shapes and sizes, wispy white curtains, the perfect towels, the perfect sheets and lots of beanbags.

At the opening, it still didn't have a name. I wasn't supposed to call it a birth center, but it was. I eventually called it Agoola, which means round in Hebrew because the living room is round; it was designed to reflect the roundness of women and their pregnant wombs.

It was 150 meters from my house; I walked to work.

Agoola was an architectural expression of everything I knew about birth. I did my best to create a soft, inspiring and natural space that would support and serve the birth process for women. I filled the closets and cabinets with fragrant soaps, oils and candles. In the kitchen, there were many kinds of coffee, a myriad of teas and spices, honey, juices, crackers and jams. I had given birth to a beautiful place, and I was in love with the baby.

The Premier

Shira was the first woman to give birth at Agoola. Both Shira and Nimrod loved the birth center from the minute they first saw it, and they were sure that this was the perfect place for them to have the perfect birth. I was excited too but things still weren't completely ready, and knowing that Shira's birth was around the corner, I was forced to quicken the pace in organizing the final details. I had been making lists for months, trying to anticipate every need that could possibly arise. Almost everything on my list was checked off except olive oil. I wanted something local and authentic.

On Sunday evening Shira and Nimrod met with Avishag at the birth center for some breastfeeding preparation. A few other couples were supposed to come, but it didn't work out. They went solo with Avishag. The meeting must have raised Shira's oxytocin levels because that night her waters broke, and she immediately went into active labor. She called me at about 3 am to let me know. It was like a dream. I got out of bed, showered, organized myself and took my bags over to the new house down the street, which was patiently waiting to witness and host its first birth experience.

They arrived a few minutes after I did, around 4:15. I had just enough time to light the salt lamps, put on some music, open the windows and get excited. I was so buzzed that I skipped drinking a cup of coffee.

They were both in great moods. We were all eager, each for his/her own reasons. They brought in their bags, checked out the house and settled in. They chose the beanbag corner; each of us was sprawled out on his/her own beanbag. They were laughing a lot and teasing each other like two puppy dogs. We drank tea and told stories. Shira's contractions were coming every four minutes, and they gradually got longer and stronger. Her mood stayed great, and the smiles and laughter never stopped.

At about 5:15, I examined Shira, and she was four cm. dilated and 100% effaced. Everything was looking good. After the exam, she went to the toilet and then into the shower. The water was soothing, and she enjoyed every minute of every contraction, the water, the tub, the presence of her adorable husband and the idea that she was doing it her way.

She decided to fill the tub and explored different positions, sitting and lying in the water as the contractions got stronger and stronger. She was breathing, relaxing, centering and using all the positive energy in the room to help her to deal with the contractions that were getting more and more impressive.

At about 6 am she was nine cm. dilated, and I called Maya. A sunrise chorus of birds was chirping outside the window of the bathroom. Shira started feeling pressure, and she pushed on and off as the urge came and went on its own. Maya happily took on her favorite role as the friendly birth photographer. At 7:10 Shai was born. Shira pushed the head out gently, guiding it with her hand as she listened to her body's cues. She asked for some help with the shoulders, and I was happy to lend a hand. Shai was born into her mother's arms as she was scooped out from below the water's surface.

Shira and Nimrod had been prepared to welcome a son into the world and were pleasantly surprised to discover a beautiful baby girl instead. She was and still is very beautiful indeed.

Shira asked for her cell phone and called her parents with the exciting news even before the placenta was out. After an ecstatic phone call, the placenta was born into the tub and scooped into a bowl and taken away for examination and storage in the freezer to be buried in the birth center garden at a later date. Everything was exactly as it was meant to be. Shira took Shai into her arms and close to her breast, and Nimrod all but jumped into the tub to be as close to them as was physically possible.

When Shira gave me the cue, I opened up the drain, and all evidence of the birth disappeared. Shira showered as Nimrod held Shai in his arms. They all gathered together in the bed, clean, happy and relieved that everything had unfolded according to the vision. They were in love with each other and with Shai who was truly a gift to all of us. A baby girl and a birth center were born simultaneously.

I left the room for a moment and cried tears of joy and relief in Maya's arms. This was a rare moment in my life in which I felt the pure euphoria of witnessing a dream coming true. I was floating. What struck me most was the simplicity of Shira's birth. If the conditions are perfect, birth can be simply beautiful or beautifully simple.

Shira's parents and her sister arrived shortly after the birth with fruits, chocolates, vegetables, cheeses, cakes and bread. They met their new granddaughter and niece, camped out together in the bedroom with Shira and Nimrod, drank coffee and ate brownies.

Later they made breakfast for all of us, and we had a birthday party in the living room. We had wine with breakfast and raised our glasses to toast the beautiful baby Shai, the amazing woman and new mother Shira, the adorable partner and new father Nimrod and a new (old) way of giving birth. The only thing that was missing was olive oil for the salad dressing.

Shira and Nimrod stayed overnight. This allowed us to talk about the joys and the challenges of what was facing them, parenthood. During the pregnancy, the focus is usually on the birth, the enormous mountain that needs to be climbed. Most first-time parents aren't aware of the entire range of mountains waiting for them on the horizon beyond the first summit.

For a first birth, this birth had been very quick, and I shared my thoughts with Shira and Nimrod about that. It was clear that her body did an amazing job, but I was concerned that maybe the rest of her needed a bit more time to adjust to the transition. This turned out to be the case. The first few months were rough for her. Shai cried a lot; the breastfeeding took time to establish itself.

It was summer, and it was hot. Shira was alone most of the time, and she felt herself slipping into a bad state. Avishag started a group for new mothers and their babies at Agoola. Once a week she fed them breakfast and provided a safe space for their questions, concerns, insecurities and feelings of isolation. Shira readily joined the group, and as a result, we saw each other once a week for months. I watched the mother in her being born, growing and developing, mountain after mountain, crisis after crisis, week by week, riding the ups and the downs. I was always proud to be her midwife.

Shira and Nimrod had two more babies with me at the birth center. She held the trophies in all the categories: she was the first woman to give birth in Agoola, the first woman to give birth there twice, and the first woman to give birth there three times. Surely, she is an honorary member of the circle of Agoola.

Lessons learned:
1. The physical environment contributes considerably to the atmosphere created at a birth.
2. A space created especially for birth contains positive energy that is sensed by everyone who enters it.
3. Even first births can be quick, simple and easy.
4. It is worthwhile to dream and to invest time, energy and resources in making dreams come true.

Michal's Two Births

Sometimes it took more than one birth to find the path to Agoola. Michal's story started with a homebirth, passed through the hospital and ended up at the birth center.

Michal and Ofir are both kibbutzniks. They have known each other since high school and have been together ever since. Michal is a nursery school teacher, has a degree in special education and is trained to work with the deaf. Ofir teaches at a school that prepares prospective university students for psychometric exams.

Michal was deeply committed to having their baby at home. It took time for Ofir to warm up to the idea, but he trusted her instincts and invested a huge amount of effort in trying to trust me. Michal and I made our initial connection in February and slowly, month by month, we got to know one another until summer came and Michal was ripe for the baby to arrive.

Contractions started on a Friday that was exactly Michal's due date. The first contractions were irregular, coming every seven to ten minutes. She and Ofir went about their business throughout the day. They bought a bouquet of white roses to inspire purity, opening and calm. In the evening the contractions started coming more frequently, at times every five minutes.

By 8 pm the intensity of the contractions increased, and their pattern was more regular; Michal asked me to come to their house. By the time I got there the contractions had become less painful, were coming every ten minutes and were gradually petering off. We listened to the baby's heartbeat, talked and decided unanimously that I should go home and wait for a call in a few hours.

The next call came at 4 am. Michal had been awake through the night with contractions lasting a minute and coming every five minutes. I showered, shook the sleep out of my body and drove back to the kibbutz. I was greeted by Ika the white Labrador Retriever who was very curious about all the unusual activity at her house in the middle of the night. Although she was sleepy and her eyes were drooping, she wasn't about to miss an event as interesting as the birth of her younger sister.

Michal behaved like a woman in early labor with contractions every five minutes, breathing and concentrating on coping with her discomfort. She wasn't concerned about her ability to handle the pain. She was tired and just wanted to sleep. She had already called her friend Ronit who was going to support her during labor, and she was on her way.

Ronit arrived at about 5:30 and brought with her all kinds of surprises and goodies. She enthusiastically massaged Michal's back, held her, spoke kind and encouraging words and used vocalization to help ease her discomfort. After sunrise, Michal and Ofir took a short walk outside and returned after 15 minutes. There were too many people on the sidewalks of the kibbutz, even so early in the morning.

Michal preferred to be in her own space inside the apartment. We closed all the curtains and shades and pushed the sunlight, the heat and the outside world away. We were in a world of our own where time had a different meaning, and the clock had a rhythm and pace of its own. We were in a different time zone known as "birth time." We listened to the music that Michal and Ofir had prepared for the birth and tasted some of the chocolates that Ronit brought.

Michal progressed slowly from 1.5 cm. at 4:50 am to three cm. at 1:40 pm. At times the contractions seemed more intense and at other times less so. Michal was in and out of the shower and the birth pool. Being in the water seemed to move the birth forward. On the other hand, the baby's position switched from occipito-anterior to occipito-posterior, and this piqued my curiosity. I was wondering what would cause a term baby of average weight to still be searching around for a good position. The possibility of a short cord or a shortened cord entered my mind. By 2:50 pm the contractions were coming every seven minutes, and it was clear to all of us that the pace of this birth was slowing down again.

It was Shabbat afternoon, and it was hot outside. After consulting with two home birth midwife friends, I suggested drinking half a glass of wine in order to allow Michal to rest and maybe even get some well-deserved and greatly needed sleep. She was hesitant, not being a wine drinker, but Ofir thought it was a great idea and Michal drank a glass of fine wine that Ofir just happened to have in the house.

She relaxed, closed her eyes and fell asleep. Ronit and I both slipped away and went home. In the car on my way home, I thought again about the possibility of a short umbilical cord not applying consistent and uniform pressure to Michal's cervix, thus causing the labor to stall over and over. There just wasn't enough momentum.

At home, I fell asleep almost immediately. Before I dozed off, I was thinking about why the labor was progressing so slowly. But sleep has its way of happening when it's needed, and thank goodness for the sleep I managed to enjoy because I woke up to Michal's phone call at 5 pm. She had rested but hadn't really slept. Her contractions were coming every four minutes and were significantly stronger. When I arrived, I checked her cervix and, lo and behold, four cm, 100% effaced, S-2. We were all elated. We had passed over a hump and felt like we were back on the path.

Michal and I had a long, quiet talk in the bedroom. She understood that she had to change her approach to the contractions. She decided that she needed to be alone and that all the tools she needed were inside of her. She didn't want her back rubbed; she didn't even want to be held. She needed only the silent presence of Ofir, and if he needed a break, she would ask that I step in. She decided not to call Ronit back to the birth. Turning each contraction into a festival had exhausted her, and she knew that it was not the right way to go.

Michal got back into the pool, and again the water seemed to nudge the labor forward. At times the contractions came every three minutes and were getting stronger. At 8:45 pm her cervix was dilated 6 cm.; the head was at S-1. Things were looking good. I started getting my equipment out in preparation to receive the baby. I was optimistic.

At about midnight Michal's cervical dilatation hadn't changed, nor at 2 am. We were over five hours at the same dilatation of 6 cm. Michal was exhausted; her mood went up and down as did her energy level. At times she seemed as if she had just begun labor and at other times, two sleepless nights seemed to be taking their toll. She dozed off in between contractions and even fell asleep sitting in the pool. We tried three doses of homeopathic Caulophyllum which got the contractions moving for about 30 minutes before they slowed down again. Ika watched over Michal throughout the labor and barely left her side.

We started thinking and talking about transferring to the hospital, even though there was no immediate cause for concern. Maybe it was just a very long, latent phase. My mind started racing, thinking about what else could be done, what had I forgotten and what recesses of possibility and wisdom remained yet unexplored.

At 1:45 am, with her permission, I ruptured Michal's waters, which were clear and plentiful, to see if that might nudge the labor along. Upon examining her I noted that the head did not come down during the contractions. There was no pressure on the cervix. After the rupture of the membranes, the contractions picked up their pace for a while and then slowed down again. I relaxed on the sofa in the living room, thinking that we were nearing the time to transfer, but I fell asleep and was awakened by Ofir calling me into the bedroom.

Ofir and Michal wanted to talk about what was happening. They both felt that the birth was going nowhere. It was almost 3 am, and we were all tired and losing our optimism that this baby would be born at home. My thoughts were confirmed when I checked her again and found a swollen cervix, the head rising and the dilation shrinking. Not only were we not going forward, but we were also starting to go backward.

Michal made one more desperate attempt to force the baby down by emphatically bouncing on the birth ball and trying to force it down, but it only made the cervix angrier. We decided to get organized and move to the hospital.

I called Bnai Zion and was greeted by a young midwife whom I had trained. A room was free, and it would be waiting for Michal. I thanked her and we were on our way. Michal's mood was at rock bottom. She was so disappointed, even though she knew that there was no point in continuing at home.

She felt that we had used all our options, and the best thing to do was to go to the hospital before the baby started suffering from this long labor. We all drove together in Ofir's car. Michal had a hard time with the contractions in the car without the motivation of the home birth. It was difficult for her to cope from a vantage point of disappointment.

On arrival, we were greeted by another former student of mine, who ushered us straight into a room without stopping in the admitting area. Many couples were waiting to be seen, heard and cared for and I was thankful for the special treatment we received. The midwife took over quickly and efficiently, filling in the forms, putting in an IV line, bringing in a consultant, starting the Pitocin drip, and calling the anesthesiologist to perform an epidural.

When the pain was taken away by the numbing effect of the epidural, Michal relaxed and Ofir fell asleep on a mattress on the floor. We talked in the dark room. After a few hours, the midwife reported a cervical dilation of seven cm., 100%, and no edema. She let me check her also just to be sure and make a comparison with what I felt before. We were back on track again. A vaginal birth was visible on the horizon.

Michal was fully dilated at 8:45 am and gave birth at 11:35. A seasoned midwife had taken over in the morning and conducted a conventional, back-lying, purple-pushing birth. Michal tried to use the knowledge she had acquired to do otherwise but was exhausted and only partially present mentally and emotionally. I passively lapsed into the role of the silent onlooking photographer.

Naomi weighed more than anyone had anticipated, 3650 grams. She was absolutely beautiful but had the shortest umbilical cord I had ever seen, less than 20 cm. When she was placed on her mother's body, it was way below her belly button because of the tug of the cord. The guilty party and the reason for the long, slow birth with the irregular contractions had been discovered. It was an extraordinarily short cord. It was a relief to have something to blame so that we could all stop blaming ourselves.

Three years later Michal became pregnant again, and we met during her 21st week. She again wanted an out-of-hospital birth; this time she wanted to give birth at Agoola instead of at their home. She was frustrated by the outcome of Naomi's birth and determined to succeed this time. Ofir was less than enthusiastic about the idea, as he was afraid that something might happen to Michal during the birth.

We negotiated with his fear and found a solution that was acceptable to everyone. When Michal entered active labor we would call an ambulance to wait outside Agoola. If we needed them, they would be right there. If they turned out to be unnecessary Ofir would pay them, say thank you and send them home. Michal was disinterested in discussing the topic but allowed Ofir to take care of the details. She had a strong, intuitive feeling that everything would be fine.

During our meetings, we discussed her previous birth experience, and Michal had two main requests. She did not want to give birth on her back, and she wanted to feel like the adult that she is, responsible and in control of her own destiny. At the hospital, she had felt like a three-year-old being told what to do, and she did not want to experience that feeling again even if we ended up transferring to the hospital. For that reason, she chose the English Nazareth Hospital as her backup plan in case the need for a hospital arose. I could continue to be her midwife and be sensitive to her needs. Ofir took care of all the arrangements with the ambulance.

At week 38 Michal discovered that she was Group B Streptococcus Positive and would need to receive IV Penicillin every four hours during the labor. At the time the home birth protocols of the Department of Health allowed for home birth midwives to administer antibiotics at home if necessary. Michal acquired the necessary prescription, the doctor's orders and the antibiotics. I supplied the equipment, the capability and the willingness to do this. We were ready.

As in her first birth, Michal felt her first contractions on her due date. Throughout the day they were irregular and not impressive enough to warrant them coming to Agoola. That night, at 3:15 am, I received a phone call from Ofir with the news that the contractions were coming every five minutes and that they would be arriving in an hour or so. I got showered and dressed and met them there at 4:30. Michal was having contractions every five minutes.

Because experience has proven that second births can be quicker than is often expected, we decided that it would be a good idea for them to come to the birth center early on to allow Michal to receive two doses of antibiotics, four hours apart, before the baby arrived. I put in the IV line and gave Michal the first and second doses at 4:40 and 8:40. In between, she and Ofir went for a walk. An hour later the contractions became stronger and close together, and her cervix was three centimeters dilated.

The birth progressed slowly and gradually throughout the day with walks, talks, contractions and antibiotics every four hours. At 4:30 pm Michal was six centimeters dilated and at 6:30 seven cm. She went into the shower. Ofir seemed a bit anxious to me. I suggested to him that he call the ambulance to wait outside the house as he had planned. After he did this, and the ambulance arrived and parked by the curb, I could feel the relaxation in his voice, his posture and his words.

Something deep inside of Michal also let go when she felt Ofir's calm. The contractions started coming every three minutes, and at 8:40 her cervix was dilated nine centimeters and the baby's head was coming down. We filled up the tub and she relaxed in the warm water. Ofir was by her side, calm and supportive.

Twenty minutes later, Michal's waters broke spontaneously, and they were clear. The contractions got even stronger, and by 9:30 she was fully dilated. She wanted to get out of the tub and onto the bed. Michal pushed her baby out on her own steam lying on her side. At 9:50 pm Amalia was cuddled in her mother's loving arms, and Michal was as happy as happy can be. When she got her wits about her, she proclaimed that it was as if her pregnancy had lasted three years, and now she felt that she had finally given birth.

After the placenta came out, Ofir thanked the ambulance crew and sent them home. They had been an important part of the support team for Ofir. Michal wasn't even aware of their presence.

Witnessing Michal's determination and participating in her victory were exhilarating experiences for me. Empowered women empower others: their spouses, their children, their parents and their midwives. Michal did her part to contribute to my belief in the power of women, babies and birth, and I thank her for this precious gift.

Lessons learned:

1. Progress in birth is affected by many factors, and it is essential to remember that 50% of them are inside the womb. When labor stalls it may be because of a fetal factor that is beyond the scope of our influence.
2. Sometimes it takes more than one attempt to get the birth you want.
3. A highly motivated woman with a clear goal is like a force of nature. You do not want to stand in her way.
4. The desire for a healing birth experience doesn't go away. It waits patiently from one birth to the next.
5. Every newborn deserves to land in the waiting arms of relaxed and loving parents.

Pizza in the Oven

Shirli came to see me early in her first pregnancy. She and her partner Ronen were excited to expand their family of three, a man, a woman and a dog, and they were happily anticipating the arrival of Sunny. They had also taken on the services of a doula, Sharon, because they were sure that they would need the support of at least two professionals. Sharon had never been at a home birth before and was a little nervous about it but agreed to join the team.

Shirli did yoga, read books, ate healthy foods and did all she could to prepare for the birth. She knew that she would want to eat Ronen's special, homemade pizzas during the birth, so in preparation, at week 38, Ronen brought to Agoola a special ceramic stone for baking pizza in the oven.

Shirli's contractions started in the early evening hours, soon after Ronen came home from work. They started becoming more frequent, and in the meantime, Ronen fell asleep on the couch. At midnight her waters broke, she woke up Ronen, and the excitement began. Sunny was on his way.

They waited a few hours at home for the contractions to become stronger, collected Sharon from her home and arrived at Agoola at about 4:30 am. The lights were low, candles were lit and music was playing in the background. The contractions were far apart, and it was still dark outside, so after I got everyone settled in, both Ronen and I fell asleep on living room couches. Sharon and Shirli were together in the bedroom doing Shiatsu. Then we switched roles, and Sharon got some sleep.

At 8 am my friend Gomer arrived to play her role in the plan as the second midwife. Because she had never been at a home birth before, we decided ahead of time that she would come from the beginning. She brought fresh energy, crackers and cheese. We were two midwives, a doula, a birthing woman, a supportive partner (and pizza chef) and a baby ready to be born.

The morning went by as Ronen prepared the pizza dough; Shirli's contractions were more or less consistent. At noon Shirli and Sharon took a long walk around the moshav, and the contractions picked up in frequency and intensity. They returned to the birth center hungry. Ronen got busy in the kitchen making pizzas for all of us.

I check Shirli, and there is no cervical dilation. Sharon prepares a vaginal steam for Shirli with rosemary branches from the garden. It works, and the contractions get stronger. Shirli gets into the bath and has her pizza delivered to the bathtub. During the contractions, Sharon holds her plate, and in between contractions she takes small bites. Sharon, Gomer, Ronen and I make sure that Shirli is never alone and that her needs are met.

At 5:30 pm her cervix is dilated three and a half centimeters. There is progress, but it is slow. I give Shirli a homeopathic remedy that I think might help, and it does. The contractions get stronger, and I am kept busy preventing Shirli from biting Ronen's finger. As evening falls, we continue to eat pizza. Shirli continues to work with the contractions, and Sharon continues to massage Shirli's legs.

At 9:30 pm she is five centimeters dilated and gets back into the bathtub. She is eight centimeters at 1 am and dilated at 5:00 am. Though it was a long night, Shirli was still determined to do this, and she took advantage of all the support she had at her disposal.

The head was low, but when she pushed it hardly budged. We tried every position and movement possible, and in good spirits, Shirli did everything Sharon, Gomer and I suggested. She was exhausted, but over and over she somehow managed to dig deeper inside herself and find more strength to go on. She started to feel the pressure of the head coming down, but it wasn't coming out. Sharon suggested using the toilet plunger to improvise a vacuum delivery. It felt good to laugh.

I hear some mild decelerations in the baby's heart rate during some of her pushing efforts. Gomer and I exchange glances; transfer to the hospital is in the air. Shirli begs us not to transfer her and reassures me that she can do this. Gomer puts in an I.V. line to increase the blood volume to the placenta in hope that it will take care of the decelerations. I put an oxygen mask on Shirli's face. Sharon is shouting in her ear, coaching her through each contraction. Ronen supports her from behind. Progress is minimal, and the decelerations continue. She has been pushing for over three hours. After I consult with Gomer, I decide to call an ambulance. Shirli begs me to let her continue pushing until they arrive.

The driver arrives with two eager, young volunteers who have never been at a birth. Shirli can feel Sunny's head, but it isn't budging. She invites the ambulance crew to join us in the room. She promises them that she can do this. They too prefer that she gives birth here and not in the ambulance. The ambulance driver is impressed with the care Shirli is receiving and tells us so more than once.

I explain to Shirli that if I cut a small episiotomy, the baby will probably come out. I do not own episiotomy scissors and am not sure how this is going to happen. Ronen assures her that this is the right thing to do, and despite her protests, I make a small snip with the scissors from the cord clamping set. Sunny rolls out and into my hands, gives a good cry and I place him into Shirli's waiting arms.

Ronen is bawling but manages to get his wits about him, enough to play the song *Sunny* by Boney M. The volunteers are crying, the ambulance driver is excited to witness a home birth, Gomer is shaking her head knowingly, Sharon is happy and relieved and I am stunned by what just happened. Never, in a million years, had I imagined a birth at Agoola with oxygen, intravenous fluids, an episiotomy and an ambulance crew.

The placenta comes out, members of the crew ask some professional questions, and I do some teaching. Shirli cuts the umbilical cord, and Ronen asks to hold his son. Shirli is ecstatic with gratitude. Everyone was thanking someone for something. I was exhausted, but I was thankful for the strength and stamina of both Shirli and Sunny, for Ronen's ability to patiently support Shirli for hours, for Sharon's help, support and cooperation, for Gomer's wisdom and guidance, for the ambulance crew, who brought a lot of positive energy into the room and for the oxygen, intravenous fluids and scissors that made it possible to complete this birth outside of the hospital. Hallelujah!

Lessons learned:

1. Women know how much support they need during birth. It is important that the expecting mother ask for and receive the amount and type of support she requires, even if it seems like too much.
2. Patience, patience, and more patience. Every birth, every woman, and every baby has its own rhythm and pace, and this uniqueness must be respected.
3. The medical equipment I carry around in my bags is there in case the need arises. I drag it back and forth, to and from every birth. I pack it into the trunk of my car before I leave the house and unpack it when I get home, rarely using it. Thanks to that equipment, this birth ended in Agoola and not in the hospital against all the odds.
4. Some birthing women enjoy the company and support of many onlookers during their labor; for them, the more the merrier works well.

Star-Crossed Mothers

Amit came to me on the recommendation of two friends of hers who had given birth with me. This was to be her second birth, and she wanted it to be better this time around even though her first birth experience was far from traumatic. She gave birth with the midwife with whom she and her husband Matan had done a birth preparation course. It was natural and relatively quick, but she remained in the hospital with her baby for five days because of mild neonatal jaundice. The breastfeeding went well, but she had a painful episiotomy to deal with.

Amit and Matan planned to have their baby at the birth center. Our first meeting was during her 32nd week; her due date was March 6. The first time around she gave birth during her 38th week, so there was a clear possibility that she could do so again, maybe around the end of February.

Amit was smart and fun. We only met three times, and our meetings were short, but I enjoyed getting to know her. She was decisive. She knew what she wanted and didn't make a fuss about anything. She warned me that she was stubborn, which didn't faze me. Stubbornness can be an advantageous quality for a woman who wants a natural birth. Her only request for this birth was to be more present and aware than at her first birth. This is a popular request for a second birth.

Amit had two concerns. She was worried about the danger of cord prolapse and wanted to know how I would handle a situation in which two women would happen to go into labor at the same time. I explained to her about cord prolapse, what it is, how it happens and how rare it is. In all my years as a midwife, I had never even seen it even once. About the possibility of two births at the same time in the birth center, I tried to calm her down by telling her that, up until then, there had been 59 births at the birth center, and two women hadn't ever gone into labor at the same time.

Efrat and Gil first came to meet me during Efrat's 31st week. This was her first pregnancy, and the idea of an out-of-hospital birth started germinating in her mind around week 29. On one hand, she didn't want to have to battle with doctors and protocols in the hospital, and she wanted to be free to direct all of her attention inward. On the other hand, she had been told that her sister had experienced a cord prolapse when she was born, a rare and terrifying experience for the mother and a life-threatening one for the baby. It was a little strange that two women due around the same dates were concerned about cord prolapse. I barely paid attention to the coincidence.

Efrat was a beautiful, confident woman. She works as a professional tour guide and has the rough, rugged and strong outward appearance of a woman who hikes a lot and knows how to take charge. Gil has two sons from a previous marriage. Efrat had a lot on her plate. Nevertheless, she seemed to be managing it all very well. She has a good relationship with Gil's sons, and they are excited about the arrival of their little brother.

Efrat and Gil decided to give birth at the birth center. Efrat's requests for the birth were that the atmosphere be relaxed, quiet and warm, without any pressure and with as little coaching as possible. She was not afraid of the pain; she felt that she had the tools to cope with it. She loves the water and planned to use the bath.

Efrat's due date was March 2, a little too close for comfort to Amit's. I figured that Amit would give birth early, and there would be plenty of time for Efrat. Statistically, first births tend to come later and tend to be longer. It would be best if Amit were to give birth early and make lots of room for Efrat, but no one has any control over all this.

At the time there was a young Canadian midwife named Ashira apprenticing with me. She had studied Midwifery in England and wanted to familiarize herself with Israeli birth culture. Ashira had been living in Agoola for several months, and she accompanied me to all my prenatal check=ups, births and postpartum visits. She slept on a sofa bed in the clinic.

Efrat called me on Feb. 26 at 10:30 am to tell me that she had experienced contractions the night before between 4-7 am. She then fell asleep and when she woke up, the contractions had calmed down. She just thought that I should know. I didn't hear from her again until the next evening, Feb. 27, at 8 pm, when she reported that her mucous plug had come out and that the contractions were back but were still irregular.

A half-hour later she called again to report that the contractions were coming every ten minutes and that they were lasting one minute. She was doing great at home, coping well with the contractions and trying to rest as much as possible in preparation for the birth which she anticipated would take place that night. I decided to go to bed early to get some sleep before Efrat's next phone call. I alerted Ashira that there would probably be a birth that night. She cleaned the kitchen and the bathrooms in preparation for guests.

The phone rang at 11:15 pm and woke me up. Nothing could have prepared me for what happened next. It was Amit on the phone, not Efrat. She was having strong contractions every six minutes. Their car was packed. She and Matan were waiting for the grandparents to arrive to be with Yuval. They would be on their way to the birth center as soon as possible.

They called from the car a few minutes after midnight. They were on their way. All I could do was hope that everything would work out, but I felt like I was about to participate in a train crash. I woke up Ashira and updated her on the surprising and somewhat terrifying turn of events.

We greeted them at the birth center at 12:40 am when they arrived. Amit was experiencing painful contractions every five minutes. Within half an hour they started coming more frequently. I examined her; her cervix was dilated five cm., and she wanted to get into the bathtub, so we filled it up. She settled in, and her body relaxed in the warm water.

At 2:20 Amit called me into the room because everything seemed to be more intense. I examined her again hoping to find a huge dilation, she was 6 cm. dilated and the head was coming down. I called Maya. I needed two more hands. I explained to Maya what was happening, and she arrived twenty minutes later ready to help in whatever way she could.

At 3:15 Efrat called to report that her waters had broken, she was having contractions every six minutes and they were getting stronger. Her amniotic fluids were clear, and she wanted to continue to stay at home. They were still waiting for Gil's parents to come to take care of his sons. This was good news because we needed just a little more time.

At 3:40 Amit's waters broke, she was having contractions every three minutes and her cervix was eight cm. dilated. At 3:45 her baby girl Noga was born into the warm water, and everything was good. Mazal tov! The placenta separated and came out spontaneously. I then told her and Matan what had been going on during the last few hours and that another woman was in active labor. We had to figure this out together.

When I planned the birth center, I kept the possibility of this scenario in the back of my mind. My clinic, also the second bedroom where Ashira was sleeping, had a sofa with a foldout bed in it. We had a plan. Instead of putting Amit in the birthing room, we would open up the sofa bed and get her settled in the clinic together with her baby and Matan. Ashira had to move all her stuff out of sight. Amit was happy and excited to be a part of all this. She understood that nothing like this had ever happened before, and she enjoyed participating in this unique and challenging situation.

We got the clinic ready for Amit, Matan and the baby by providing soft lights, clean sheets, a nursing pillow and a pot of hot tea. Matan moved their bags in while Ashira moved her things out. Maya and I moved Amit and the baby. Maya got them settled while Ashira and I started cleaning. After they were settled in and the baby was nursing, we closed the door. There was no trace of the birth that had just occurred. It was as if they had never even been there.

We changed the sheets, gathered the dishes into the kitchen sink, sterilized the bathtub and the toilet, and washed the floor. Everything was put back in place. Maya and Ashira jokingly asked if they could measure my blood pressure. I agreed, and I shudder when I recall the numbers that I saw flashing before my eyes on the BP machine. It is a miracle that I didn't have a heart attack or a stroke.

At 4:50 Efrat called to say that the contractions were coming every four minutes and that they were getting ready to come. Everything was clean and ready to go. We drank a cup of coffee and waited for them to arrive.

They walked in at 5:20. Efrat's face was flushed, she was having contractions every three minutes and she was delighted to be in active labor. The three of us stood near the front door and received Efrat and Gil like a bride and groom. I examined her and found a cervical dilation of nine cm. The head was low and pressing down powerfully. This baby was pushing his way out.

Twenty minutes later she was fully dilated, and fifteen minutes after that, her baby boy Alon was cuddled safely in her arms. She never made it into the nice, clean bathtub; she gave birth on the bed. The placenta came out ten minutes later, and we all sighed a huge sigh of relief. Efrat got settled in bed with her baby and her adoring husband. We then told Efrat and Gil that there was another couple with a brand-new baby in the next room. It didn't phase them.

Nobody seemed to care. No one was upset about the lack of privacy or the need to share the facility. No one cared that this could have worked out badly. Nobody seemed to have a problem with anything. It was a bit surreal.

And then the party began. First, the husbands met in the kitchen and made more tea for their wives. Then they started talking, getting to know each other and getting comfortable with the situation. One thing led to another, and by the morning, the four of them were preparing and eating breakfast together.

When I finished documenting both births, I realized that they are neighbors and live on the same street in Tivon.

These two babies grew up and went to the same nursery school. Their parents became friends and remained so for many years. Three years after the magical night, both Amit and Efrat got pregnant again, and this time they had exactly the same due date. Both gave birth with me again. Fortunately, this time there was one whole day between the two births.

Something about their destiny is connected. Maybe Noga and Alon will remain good friends and marry one another someday. Who knows? I know that as long as I live, I will never forget that night. I could feel Fate smiling down on all of us, and it felt amazing.

Lessons learned:

1. I need to trust, believe and let go. This was the only way that I could possibly cope with this situation, which at first seemed impossible and turned out to be magical.
2. The Universe has a sense of humor. It's a good idea to learn to laugh along with it.
3. Worrying is a terrible waste of energy. Reality is nothing like the catastrophes we create in our minds. I saw a train wreck in my mind, and it turned into a roller coaster ride.

Closing and Opening the Doors

When I planned and built Agoola, I kept in the back of my mind the thought that one day one of my children might want to make it their home.

It functioned as my clinic and birth center for four years, during which time sixty-three women began their births. Six transferred to hospitals; fifty-seven gave birth in the birth center. They brought healthy, sweet babies into the world with no dressing gowns, IV lines (except Shirli) or monitor straps. There was no rushing; there were no strangers, no threats and no lies. I welcomed thirty-two water babies into the tub designed exactly for that purpose.

Mothers labored on the floor, the birth chair, the bed, in the shower, on the toilet, in the kitchen, on their knees, on all fours, sitting, standing, squatting, side-lying and on their backs. No two births were alike, just as no two women are alike, no two couples are alike and no two moments are alike.

The birth center allowed me the freedom to work in an atmosphere of professional autonomy, unlike anything else I had ever experienced anywhere. And then Agoola closed its doors to birthing couples for the best of reasons.

My son Eitan and his wife Naama announced that they were expecting a baby in September 2011 and that they wanted to leave their apartment in Tel Aviv and move into Agoola. With this announcement, they were also proclaiming that Eitan would be moving back to the village of his childhood, we were about to become grandparents, they were to become our neighbors and all of our lives were about to change forever.

Agoola would cease to exist as a birth center; it would become the home of my son, my daughter-in-law and my grandchildren. The birth center would need to move, and luckily, an alternative space was available. There was a living unit on the lower level of our house that had housed my parents when they used to visit. It needed a renovation, and we got to work.

The bathroom was gutted; new ceramics, a new shower, a new toilet and a big, beautiful, deep, wide bathtub were installed. Shelves were built, a soundproof door installed and some walls constructed to create a feeling of privacy and safety. The final act was to paint the walls with the same lovely color that made Agoola feel so warm and welcoming.

"Operation Move Agoola" required precision planning because several women were due, and I couldn't allow for a gap between the two locations. A phone call from a woman with contractions could shake my world at any moment. In order to be able to fall sleep at night, I needed to know that we could move the furniture, books, linens and kitchen supplies, hang pictures, clean up after moving and be open for business, all between sunrise and sunset of the same day.

Eitan promised me that he would make it happen; he loves logistical challenges. With a lot of help from many people, it happened one hot day in July. One door closed, and so many more opened. Agoola #2 was open for business. Naama and Eitan spent the rest of the summer settling into Agoola #1 and turning it into their new nest.

Ayelet's Three Births

Ayelet is a strikingly beautiful woman, inside and out. She has a full head of perfect, tiny black curls and a body that reflects years of exercise and good nutrition.
Her partner Dror is a sweet man and a great dad, hardworking and inventive. All three of their children were born at the birth center.

Regaining Faith in Her Body

Ayelet and Dror underwent fertility treatments for several years before she finally got pregnant for the first time with Romi. They invested an enormous energy, time and money in the process. For Ayelet, the pregnancy was filled with all the repercussions of fertility treatments: loss of self-esteem, anxiety, frustration, loss of control and loss of belief in her body. Even though she toyed with the idea of a home birth, in order to feel safer, they decided to have the baby with me in the hospital in Nazareth. Eitan and Naama had moved into Agoola #1, and so far no one had given birth in the new birth center.

I first became aware of the fact that Ayelet's birth had started when she called me first thing in the morning with strong contractions. I told them to come over so I could examine her before we left for the hospital. She was clearly in active labor, and her cervix was eight centimeters dilated. We were all pleasantly surprised.

She made an immediate and spontaneous decision to stay at the birth center. There was no way she was getting back into the car with contractions so strong and so close together. Full dilation happened pretty quickly, but it took a while for the baby to come down and out. I was glad for the time. It gave me a chance to figure out the logistics of receiving a baby in the new space.

Maya joined us, along with Ayelet's mother and sister. We all gathered around her on the bed, and when Romi was born there wasn't a dry eye in the house. There were tears of relief, joy, love and victory. She gave birth under her own steam, and it was a huge conquest for her. After being so disempowered by the fertility process, she reclaimed her power with a home birth.

It was a poignant opening for the new birth center, and there was a lot of hugging afterward.

Lessons learned:

1. Pregnancies after fertility treatments are considered high risk because so much has been invested in them. These women are seen as fragile and are treated like glass figurines. They are offered elective C-sections to circumvent birthing altogether. Ayelet refused to be categorized in this manner and proved to herself that a good, physiological birth at home could empower her and renew her belief in her body.
2. Ayelet's soul wanted to give birth at home. Her body did the work and made the dream come true. Deep desire can inspire miracles.
3. Sometimes we have a thought in our minds that something is dangerous, but our bodies tell us otherwise. We learn that what we thought was dangerous turns out to be safe. It pays to listen and learn lessons from the body.

A Premie in Agoola

Shai was also a successful product of fertility treatments. His birth began like Romi's, first thing in the morning, with strong contractions. But this time there was a catch. Ayelet was only 34+5 weeks pregnant, and she had been sick with a bad cough for two weeks.

I explained to her on the phone that we would have to go to the hospital because the baby is premature; their job was to decide which hospital. I quickly showered and got dressed. The plan was for them to pick me up and drive together to Rambam.

I had my bag on my shoulder when they pulled into my driveway. The car door opened, and Ayelet popped out of the car. She wanted me to check her because she felt like the baby was coming. We went into the birth center, and I checked her. She was right, again eight centimeters with the head pushing its way out. Again we made a quick decision to stay and have the baby at the birth center. We agreed to call an ambulance just to be on the safe side because the baby was premature.

Shai was born before the ambulance arrived and weighed almost three kilograms. He nursed immediately, and Ayelet hung on to him like a mama bear. The ambulance driver and crew waited outside while she nursed him, dressed him, took a shower and got dressed. I made them fresh coffee, and they drank it in the sun, waiting patiently. The atmosphere was lovely.

They transported all of us to Rambam to the delivery room to be admitted and processed. Shai was then moved to the Neonatal Intensive Care Unit because he was premature. He remained hospitalized for two weeks. When Ayelet first saw him in the NICU, a new kind of hell for her began.

The NICU was one of the most challenging experiences Ayelet has ever had to endure. She was sick with pneumonia and received IV antibiotics in the obstetric ward for a few days. She was weak, postpartum and devastated by being separated from her baby Shai.

Several times each day, she made her way to the children's hospital where the NICU was located. It was impossible to know what surprises awaited her each time she arrived to be with her baby. She wondered what he was doing there after all. He was bigger, hungrier and louder than any other baby there by a long shot. It all seemed so unreal. She was plagued with thoughts that all this suffering was unnecessary.

The noise of the machines, the buzzers and the monitors drove her crazy. Nurses cared for, fed, bathed and held him. There was no privacy, no intimacy and very few opportunities to express a mother's love for a newborn baby.

I visited them there and was devastated by Ayelet's distress. The NICU was a dense jungle of beeping monitoring machines, technicians, equipment, staff and sick babies. It was a sensory nightmare and navigating it was almost impossible. After two weeks they went home and tried to rehabilitate themselves and their relationship. To this day Ayelet is still working to reduce the distance she feels between herself and Shai.

Lessons learned:
1. Newborn babies should not be separated from their mothers unless one of their lives is endangered. The damage done by this disconnection is significant and has long-lasting effects. We must find a better way to take care of babies born a few weeks early that does not entail separating them from their mothers.
2. Hospitalization in the NICU can be a traumatic experience for the entire family. The parents of premature and sick babies need the kind of support that maintains their sense of safety and control while simultaneously encouraging the development of their connection with their babies.

Three is a Lucky Number

Ayelet got pregnant again, this time on her own. No plans or intentions, no medical procedures, injections or interventions. She and Dror were stunned. At first, they asked themselves whether or not they even wanted another child. But this baby came on its own power. How could they be anything but ecstatic and welcome him into their family?

It was a confusing time, but they decided to continue the pregnancy and keep the baby. When we first met it was obvious that Ayelet needed some therapy. She felt that her relationship with Shai had been damaged by his time in the NICU and couldn't talk about it without bursting into tears.

We met only three times, but her mindset changed significantly. We devoted our first meeting to exploring her resources, and she experienced the physical manifestation of feeling resourced for the first time. Both of Ayelet's parents are psychotherapists, and she has been through a lot of therapy in her life. She is also very familiar with bodywork: training, dancing, running. But she reported to me with a huge smile on her face that this was the first time she could feel, through the sensations of her body, what it actually felt like to be resourced. She was very thankful for the revelation. She went home with the understanding that she needs to spend more time doing things that make her feel good and that this could seriously affect her attitude toward her children, her husband, her pregnancy and her life. We were both optimistic.

During our second meeting, we started working on the NICU experience. We began with the birth, which provided her with a beautiful, comfortable memory of Shai nuzzled tight on her chest, of the kind and patient ambulance personnel, the ride to Rambam, and even being admitted to the delivery room. Even when Shai was taken away by the pediatrician from the NICU, she felt confident that he was in good hands.

When Dror took her down there for the first time, and she saw Shai naked under the lights, exposed and helpless, connected to tubes and wires, she received a shock to her system. There was so much distance between them; she couldn't hold him; she could barely touch him because she didn't have the strength to stand because of her pneumonia. And when she sat down, she couldn't reach him.

The sense of loss was overwhelming. There were so many losses all at once: the loss of intimacy, the loss of control, the loss of normalcy, the loss of safety and the loss of contact with the baby she had nourished in her womb for eight months. Her stomach was tightly clenched, her breath lost its natural rhythm and tears poured down her cheeks.

And the worst part of this scene was the NOISE: the buzzers, the alarms, the monitors and the nurses talking constantly in loud voices. She felt that the noise was making her dizzy, forcing her to lose her balance and lose herself.

We returned to the memory of the birth center. She seemed to be swept away by the dizziness and the noise of the NICU. In the birth center it was quiet; the only sound she heard was Shai's newborn baby cooing. Slowly Ayelet got her center back and feeling centered we went back to the NICU, but this time the power was in her hands (actually in her mind). She imagined the changes she would make to help herself feel better.

The first thing she did was to imagine turning down the volume of the nurses' voices. She imagined disconnecting all the wires from Shai's body. She took him into her arms and, together with Dror, went into the breastfeeding room so they could be alone. Ayelet sat on the oversized, comfortable lounger and held Shai close to her chest. No one bothered them; there were no interruptions and time had no meaning. It was as if they were together in a big pink bubble. She took this feeling home with her.

During our third meeting, we continued our work on the topic of the NICU. There was still considerable pain in her memories, but in addition to the pain, she was also able to see the gifts. The sources of her pain were: loss of control and privacy, wondering and doubting whether or not the treatments Shai received were even necessary, wondering how it would have been if he hadn't been premature, and not being in charge of her own son's care and not speaking up when things didn't feel right. The gifts were: her strong connection with Shai, Dror's total commitment to her and the baby, the few sacred moments of intimacy they had together, the fact that they survived the ordeal and a newly discovered ability to let go of her need for control. She was happy that the NICU exists for the sake of genuinely sick babies, and even though she felt that Shai had been over-treated, she could forgive, dismiss it and go on with her life.

Ayelet had some serious contractions at 34 weeks, and it looked as if she was going into premature labor again and would have to cope with the hospitalization of another baby in the NICU. She was confident that she could handle it, and we calmly discussed which hospital would be the best choice for them this time.

I also raised the possibility that this was a manifestation of Anniversary Syndrome, and with a warm bath, a glass of wine and a bottle of water, all this might pass. And so, it did. The contractions went away. She was tired and felt heavy, but she managed to hold on for a few more weeks. We spoke every few days, and I was optimistic that she would hold on to the pregnancy.

When she was 37+2 weeks, Ayelet woke up at about 4 am with a few painful contractions and light bleeding. She called me primarily because of the bleeding. The contractions were only every 15-20 minutes apart. She and Dror came over so I could take a look, and she was behaving like a woman in active labor. Even though the contractions were far apart, they were painful. The bleeding was minimal, but her blood pressure was high so we considered going to the hospital.

I decided to check her vaginally. The thought went through my head that this time she couldn't possibly be eight centimeters dilated with contractions so far apart. And much to my surprise, she was eight centimeters dilated (again)! And again, we decided to stay put. Ayelet didn't want to take a chance that she might give birth in the car on the way to the hospital.

We filled the bathtub with warm water, and she settled in. The contractions continued to come every 10-15 minutes, and she progressed to nine centimeters. Only during the last half hour of the birth did the contractions come every five minutes. She gave birth to her beautiful baby boy Yahli in the water, and everything was perfect. She didn't let that baby out of her arms for a minute. She gave birth as she had planned, in her own time, at her own pace, in her special way, on her own steam.

Lessons learned:

1. I try to comprehend the enormous range of rhythms possible in births. How many ways are there to give birth? The possibilities are infinite even for the same woman.
2. As long as I continue to do this work I will continue to be surprised. It is part of what draws me in.
3. In some ways, I know this work very well. Still, I sometimes feel that I know absolutely nothing at all.

The Birth of a Baby, a Mother, and a Grandmother

Early in her pregnancy, my daughter-in-law Naama and my son Eitan sat me down on our front lawn and told me they were planning a home birth, and they wanted me to be their midwife. I was shocked, ecstatic, terrified and felt a thousand other emotions simultaneously. I clearly remember the first thought that went through my mind. The budding grandmother in me came forward cautiously and said, "Home birth – isn't that DANGEROUS?" I got over myself quickly and agreed to take them on as clients. Before that beautiful baby girl was born, that grandmother would show up a few more times and ask some very silly questions.

Naama's pregnancy was eventless. They lived in Tel Aviv during most of it. Naama worked at a health food store, and Eitan was studying jewelry design. When they moved to the moshav, she was in full bloom. The three of us met regularly in my clinic for childbirth preparation, and they took a Hypnobirthing course together. She read books, watched movies, swam, did yoga, meditated and took a lot of long walks. We were all very open and honest with one another. We worked hard to keep the potential complexity of the situation in clear view.

On one hand, delivering my grandchild at home would be the peak of my midwifery career. What could be more fulfilling than that? On the other hand, I knew a lot about what could go wrong. I knew that we could end up with a transfer, a C-section or even worse. Sometimes it scared the shit out of me, and other times I reassured myself that there was a very good chance that everything would be fine. Naama was healthy, happy and active. She ate amazingly well, and she had my lovely son to support her. She had prepared well and wasn't afraid of the pain. She had faced challenges in her life, both physical and emotional and had overcome them. She was confident.

Naama and Eitan chose Lihi as their backup midwife. They met with her and felt comfortable in her presence. We planned to call her whenever we needed her, and she would join us for the second stage.

She was honored and excited to be a part of our life event.

Naama felt her first contractions on Friday morning, and toward noon they started getting more regular. It was raining, a bit unusual for September in Israel. The weather was cool and overcast. She asked me to come to the house, so I did. I walked down the street with my Doppler in hand. I was so excited that I could barely breathe. The street was empty; no one could see my flushed face or feel my body pulsing.

I found her in the living room – standing, walking, sitting on the birth ball and breathing through the contractions that were coming every five minutes. There was music, a pot of tea, a clean house and my son lovingly attending to her every need. I tried to be both present and nonobtrusive.

As the afternoon slowly turned into evening, the rain and the contractions gradually intensified. I went home to get my equipment and the car, updated Avner and called Naama's parents. They planned to come to our house to be with Avner and wait to become grandparents together.

At 6 pm we did the first internal exam. Naama's cervix was four centimeters dilated and fully effaced, but the head was high. The baby wasn't small, and Naama's hips are narrow. Throughout the pregnancy, I worried about whether the baby's head would be able to negotiate her pelvis.

She tried to open up and let the baby's head come down using movement, relaxation, determination and love. The warm bath water also helped. At 10 pm, much to my relief, the head was down, she was six centimeters dilated and the contractions were coming every three minutes. With mildly trembling fingers, I updated everyone via text messages.

The rest of the birth is mostly a blur. Luckily, I wrote some notes; otherwise, I wouldn't have remembered anything. I floated in and out of various roles, sometimes Eitan's proud mother, sometimes the professional midwife, sometimes Naama's respectful mother-in-law and sometimes the worried and expectant grandmother. I was caught in a whirlwind of emotions. I tried to ground myself as much as possible, so I could do the job I was expected to do.

At around midnight Naama's waters broke; she was eight centimeters dilated, and the head had come down. It felt like the baby was pushing her way out. I called Lihi and excitedly asked her to join us. The birth seemed imminent; she was on her way.

I called the house to update the other grandparents who were watching TV, biting their fingernails and dozing off. Both of Naama's parents are medical professionals, and they waited anxiously for frequent and detailed updates. They were thrilled at the good news. Naama got back into the tub, this time with Eitan. The warm water soothed her body and spirit.

It took another two hours for Naama to transition to full dilation. The baby's heartbeat was strong and reassuring every time I listened; she was fine. But these two hours were clearly the most difficult hours of the birth for everyone involved. Naama was in a good deal of pain, and Eitan did everything in his power to help her to cope, but I was getting ready to throw in the towel and go home. I was emotionally drained. Lihi arrived, and I asked her to take over for me. She instructed me to go outside, breathe some fresh air, and encouraged me to return when I was ready. She reassured me that I would be fine. I needed to hear that because I wasn't sure.

I could feel Naama's pain, and I could feel Eitan's need to make it better. I was over-involved emotionally and had lost my professional perspective. Also, the grandmother in me was worried for no good reason, but after all, she IS a grandmother. That is her prerogative.

When I came back into the house and the bathroom, I could feel the midwife reenter my body as I pushed the grandmother aside. Everything was fine; everyone was good. All we needed was patience and time for the head to mold itself, for the pelvic bones to open up and for sweet Noga to plow her way out into the world.

It took another two hours for this miracle to happen, and at 4:08 Noga fought her way into the world. Her head slipped out into the water, but her shoulders were stuck. They released themselves from the confines of Naama's pelvis as she stood up and raised one leg on the tub's rim. Naama became a mother, Eitan became a father and the midwife in me was proud to bear witness to this miracle. The grandmother was out of sight weeping from joy and relief in the corner somewhere.

After the placenta came out, Naama got washed off and settled into bed with Noga and Eitan. Noga crawled her way to the breast, pushed herself into a comfortable position, and took the nipple immediately into her luscious mouth. It was difficult to pull myself away, but there were three other grandparents down the street anxiously awaiting the good news.

They were at the door within a minute, beaming with joy and relief. A birthday party manifested itself in the bedroom. As Avner held me tight, I felt myself allowing some of the tension to drain out of my body. I caught a glimpse of myself in the mirror and barely recognized the woman with all the new gray hairs.

Lessons learned:

1. I have many voices inside of me. I need to allow them to express themselves.
2. Emotional entanglement at this level is challenging. It is not a good idea to be alone. At Naama's second birth I asked Lihi to join us a lot earlier.
3. Seeing the birth through my son's eyes enabled me to better understand the difficulty the partner faces during birth. I could see his strong desire to help his wife, and even more so, I could feel the frustration in his body being fueled by his inability to take her pain away.
4. The magnitude of the emotional challenge of this birth surprised me. It almost knocked me over. Afterward, I thought that nothing could be more difficult than this and that if I could do this, I could do anything.

Face to Face

Noa and Yaacov came to meet me when Noa was in the 27th week of her third pregnancy. They lived in a community called Rotem, south of Beit She'an in the Jordan Valley. It is 45 minutes from the nearest hospital and over an hour's drive from my place. They planned to have this baby at my birth center and had no expectations that I would come to their house. Noa's first two births had been positive experiences and were pretty straightforward. One was at a hospital and one at a birth center that had closed its doors. She gave birth to both boys standing up; her second stages were quick and relatively easy.

Yaacov was a large man with a burly black beard who made big babies. Both of their sons weighed around four kilograms when they were born. He worked as a tour guide and was very knowledgeable about plants, animals, history and people. Noa was gentle and soft-spoken. She worked with mother-baby dyads and was studying to become a doula. She already had substantial experience accompanying women to births. From the moment we met, I felt I was in the presence of two young people who harbored wisdom far beyond their years.

Noa's pregnancy wasn't straightforward. She had issues with her thyroid gland, an umbilical hernia, anemia and polyhydramnios. She was busy with her work and preoccupied with raising two rambunctious boys. She didn't have much free time to connect with the fetus whose sex remained unknown. During the last month and a half, she changed her nutrition and only ate raw food. She also treated herself via a healing modality called "Life Alignment" to reduce the amount of amniotic fluid and balance her thyroid functions. "Life Alignment" aims to facilitate healing, transformation, growth and consciousness by bringing the energy fields of the physical, emotional, mental and spiritual bodies back into alignment.

It worked; by the time the birth started, all her health issues had resolved themselves. Even her glucose levels were normal, and there was no evidence of gestational diabetes. This needed to be ruled out because of two big babies and the polyhydramnios. Noa's birth plan included her desire to be in the water, to be mostly alone, to give birth on Shabbat and to come to my place early in labor. She also warned me that she tends to be very sensitive to the energy of those around her.

From week 37, Noa was experiencing contractions on and off, but they didn't morph into active labor until week 39. Noa and her family were visiting with her parents on Shabbat, and it was the perfect time to have a baby. They were closer to the birth center geographically; the grandparents could be with the boys and it felt right. On Saturday morning the contractions began, and by 2 pm they were more regular, prolonged and painful. At 3 o'clock Noa called to tell me that she and Yaacov were on their way because the contractions were coming every five minutes. When they arrived at 3:45 Noa's contractions were irregular and far apart.

They went for a walk, rested, ate and watched a movie. Gradually the contractions started getting stronger and closer together. At 6:15 I examined Noa's cervix, and it was funnel-shaped, open to two cm on the outside and five cm inside, and the head was high, barely touching the cervix. The contractions weren't painful, so Noa continued to rest and enjoy a back massage from Yaacov. Eventually, she drifted off and fell asleep.

At 1:30 am she woke up with more painful contractions that were coming every five minutes. By 3:30 they were getting stronger and more significant. Noa got into the tub, and at 4:30 I examined her again and found a cervical dilation of nine cm. The head was still very high, the sac was bulging through the cervix and it was filled with amniotic fluid. This was a potentially dangerous situation that could result in the prolapse of the umbilical cord. The baby's head was hardly touching the cervix. If her waters broke, emersion in the water might lower the danger by reducing the pull of gravity on the cord.

Because of the shape of Noa's belly, the location of the fetal heart rate and the high head, I suspected that the baby was occipito-posterior, with its back in the direction of Noa's back instead of toward the front wall of her abdomen. This would also account for the irregular contractions and the slow progress. I shared with Noa and Yaacov everything I knew. Noa was now in a lot of pain, and she was feeling a lot of pressure even though the baby's head was still high. I called Maya and asked her to join us.

At 6:00 Noa left the tub and sat on the birth ball. She tried to get the head to move down by swinging her hips and bouncing on the ball. When she stood up, her waters broke, flooding the room. I immediately examined her to rule out cord prolapse. There was no cord, and I found the head, but something was odd. It wasn't smooth, round and hard. It was softer, and in the middle, something felt like a button, a tiny bulge, a protrusion. It was a nose! The baby was in a face presentation.

I fished around in an attempt to find the mouth, trying to be careful not to poke the eyes, and then I felt the tip of my finger being sucked by a tiny mouth. The mouth was in the direction of Noa's left side, for me "3 o'clock" or in obstetric/midwifery lingo, "left mento-transverse" (mento refers to the chin). Her cervix was now eight cm. dilated. I pulled my hand out. We needed to talk.

I explained to Noa and Yaacov that we were in a very odd and precarious situation. Face presentation is infrequent and it usually ends in a C-section, especially if the chin turns in the direction of the mother's back. There is no way a baby can negotiate its mother's pelvis in that position. For now, it was facing sideways and could go either way. We could either go to the hospital or wait and see. Noa decided to wait and see. If the chin would turn in the direction of Noa's pubic bone, a vaginal birth would still be possible.

We were all sailing in uncharted territory, and we all felt the tension in the air. The baby was not in danger, but this birth was not within the realm of normal. Noa asked Maya and me to stop talking about how unusual the situation was. She tried to center herself and normalize the situation. We respected her wishes and kept quiet.

All of a sudden, she had an idea. She asked Yaacov to get her Life Alignment tools, a pendulum and cards, from her bag and bring them to her. She sat alone with her tools, connected with the baby in her womb, felt her presence, strength and optimism, and she knew that everything would be okay.

At 7:40, the chin turned part way, in the right direction, toward her pubic bone. Noa got back into the tub. At 9:00, she was fully dilated, the chin had made the full turn to mento-anterior and the head was moving down. Noa left the tub, moved back to the bedroom, found a comfortable position and started pushing.

At 9:31 her beautiful baby girl came into the world, safely in her mother's waiting arms. Her face was a bit swollen and bruised, and she seemed a bit tired, but she was strong and healthy. It had been quite a journey, and she was ready to face the world.

Lessons learned:

1. This birth was a wild ride. No doubt about that. But, for me, this birth story is not about the difficulty but trust. It is about trusting the mother, the baby, the birth and myself to know what is safe and what is not.
2. The true heroine of this story is the baby girl who some day will grow up and become one very powerful woman.
3. Connection, relaxation and optimism made all the difference in this birth. Their power and influence on the birth process should not be underestimated.

178 | Birth Days

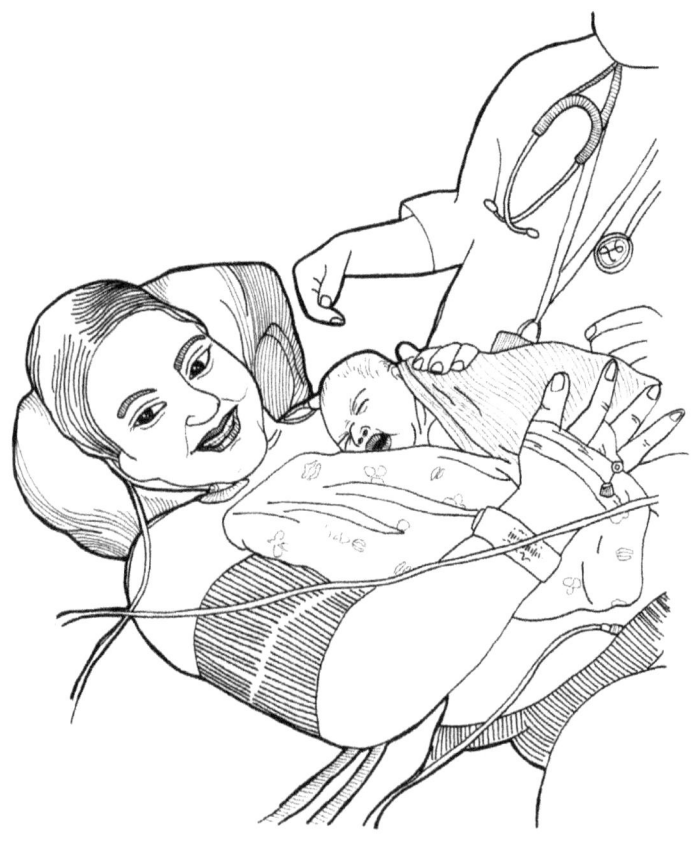

Finding a Better Way – The VBAC Heroines

VBAC (pronounced vee'-bak) is an acronym coined by Nancy Wainer Cohen, a midwife from Boston who wrote the book *Silent Knife – Cesarean Prevention and Vaginal Birth after Cesarean (VBAC)* together with Lois Estner in 1983. *The Wall Street Journal* touted it as the bible of Cesarean prevention. Its publication was viewed as an event that would change the course of obstetric care forever. It was awarded Best Book in the field of Health and Medicine by the American Library Association the year it was published. Doris Hare wrote, "Obstetricians would be wise to read this book before their patients get their hands on it."

The VBAC revolution was happening in America while I was having my babies in the 1980s. By the time I became a midwife in 1995 it was still in its early stages of taking hold in Israel. Trends take about 10-15 years to cross the Atlantic Ocean and the Mediterranean Sea to get from America to Israel. Women were still being told "Once a Cesarean, always a Cesarean" and were being scared by their Ob/Gyns into repeated and often unnecessary surgery.

I met many of these women in the delivery room in their dire attempts at a normal birth after having undergone abdominal surgery to bring their babies into the world. The odds were pitted against them from the start because of a general lack of trust in the stamina of uterine scars. Everyone was afraid of dehiscence, the splitting open of the scar left on the uterus after a Cesarean Section.

The actual incidence of scar dehiscence was only about 0.5%, and slowly the approach toward birthing women after C-sections evolved. Gradually, VBAC became the hesitant but official recommendation. And because the number of primary C-sections was skyrocketing, the number of VBACs was also rising.

To this day VBAC-ers are still modern-day heroines. They have many natural enemies lurking in the delivery rooms. There is still a lot of fear and trepidation around these births. The acronym has been changed to TOLAC – Trial of Labor After Cesarean, implying that this is only an attempt and the outcome will determine if the trial was a success or a failure.

Some doctors still encourage their clients to choose elective surgery as an option. Many women are willing to go against the recommendations of their doctors to claim back their bodies and their births. I was honored to meet and work closely with some of these brave women.

Many of them achieved their goal of birth vaginally the second time around. Unfortunately, some didn't, and they found themselves again on the operating table, in the same position, having their babies removed from their wombs surgically. My job was to help them clean the slate emotionally, guide them through the maze of options and hold on to the knowledge that healing is a real and imminent possibility.

With Her Head Held High – Ma'ayan

Ma'ayan was the survivor of one of those disastrous births in the hospital when everything that can go wrong does, and the birthing woman pays a terrible price. She was referred to me by her lactation consultant with the hope that I would accompany her to her next birth at Carmel Hospital. It wouldn't work out that way. I had planned to be abroad at the time of her birth, so we would work together until I left.

At the time Ma'ayan had a two-year-old daughter whom she described as a fighter. She knows what she wants and how to get it and is stubborn about having her needs met. She was born at one of the hospitals in Haifa in an emergency C-section after 15 hours in the natural birthing suite and several failed attempts at vacuum extraction.

When she was born, she was floppy and blue and required resuscitation. She was later put on a respirator in the NICU. A significant caput, a swelling under the scalp, was discovered behind her left ear, the sign of an apparent asynclitic presentation; her baby had entered the birth canal off-side. She was in the NICU for two days and then moved over to the healthy newborn unit before going home with her mother.

After the birth, Ma'ayan had some physical wounds to deal with. She had an episiotomy, which was cut in anticipation of the vacuum delivery. She was left with a broken rib due to repeated fundal pressure. She had a sore and injured throat as a result of emergency intubation in a crash C-section with general anesthesia. And then, of course, she had the wounds of the C-section itself.

Her emotional wounds were enormous in addition to the physical ones. She sat on my couch and cried for almost two hours, her big blue eyes filling up with tears over and over again; each time she was reminded of another source of her pain. I held on to myself for dear life, trying not to burst into tears as well.

The following is a list of everything that happened to her:

Numerous vacuum attempts were made by two different doctors, together with significant fundal pressure, also called the Kristeller maneuver. She remembers protesting, saying that she couldn't breathe and that they were hurting her. The doctors ignored her protests.

One of the female doctors screamed at her; she told Ma'ayan she was neither pushing hard enough nor cooperating. She remembers asking herself at the time, "Why is this woman taking her frustrations out on me?" At the same time, she doubted herself and wondered whether or not she was giving it her all. She felt guilty for not doing her part.

She ushered her husband out of the room before the first vacuum attempts. No one spoke to him or sought him out. Eventually, he mustered up the courage to ask what was going on and was told that his wife had already given birth by C-section and that the baby was in the NICU. In between, he was given no information or support by any staff member.

Ma'ayan remembers being "thrown" from the bed in the delivery room onto a gurney and almost falling off. She felt like an object, a piece of meat.

She did not remember being emotionally supported by any of the midwifery staff. The only person who came to her and the baby's defense was the anesthesiologist. He chastised the doctor who considered making another attempt at a vacuum extraction in the operating room. He told her to stop before she killed the baby.

After the operation was over and she understood what had happened, she wanted to see her but couldn't because she was in NICU. No one told her what the baby's condition was. No one brought in her husband to be with her. She lay in bed alone with the nurse in the recovery room and cried.

The next day it took hours before anyone tried to help her meet her baby. Eventually, she was brought to her for a few minutes and then taken away again.

The head of the department approached her, and she believes that it was only because he learned that she is a lawyer. He defended every one of the actions taken by the doctors and offered no apology, sympathy, empathy or compassion for all her suffering.

She reported to the staff that she was having trouble breathing and suspected a broken rib. No doctor dealt with this complaint or even ordered an X-ray.

Sitting up and moving around to pump colostrum was an almost superhuman task with pain coming from so many different directions.

She wanted more than anything in the world to hold, comfort and feed her baby girl, whom she felt she had abandoned.

We talked and talked, and Ma'ayan cried and cried. We tried to make some sense of the events. She asked very good questions and tried to clarify tidbits of verbal and visual memories that she had been trying to piece together for over two years. Together we tried to understand why the baby had become stuck, what was the meaning of the strangely located swelling on the baby's head, why her husband was ushered out of the room, why the doctor was so obsessed with succeeding with the vacuum and why her husband received no information.

I was curious to understand if she was feeling guilty, whether she was accusing others of being at fault, how her husband was handling this and where she stood today, pregnant and facing another birth experience. She was still angry, but parts of her contained and even accepted what had happened. She felt forgiveness for herself, her husband and the staff of the delivery room.

These were the lessons she learned from the experience:

Doctors and midwives are human. They can and will make mistakes.

She would have liked to have been able to speak up for herself and her baby but wasn't capable of doing so at the time. In preparation for this next birth, she wants to be able to defend herself and communicate more assertively.

The system isn't perfect, and its objectives are different from those of the individual.

She is not interested in continuing to be a passive, accommodating woman. She is now in search of discovering what it is she wants and no longer intends to act in ways that focus on pleasing others.

She does not want to dwell on negative thoughts and negative feelings. It weakens her. She wants to concentrate on herself and her family and on becoming happier and stronger for her own sake and theirs.

With the time we had available, we worked together on these issues. I remember Ma'ayan as an extraordinarily courageous woman. This was most evident in the manner in which she faced her traumas head-on. She was determined to feel better and not to let this horrific experience define her for the rest of her life.

After I returned from my trip abroad, I learned that Ma'ayan achieved her VBAC at Carmel Hospital. The staff was super-supportive and helped her every step along the way. She saw her second birth as a corrective experience, which allowed her to feel stronger and happier and enabled her to get back in touch with her body and herself.

My lessons learned:

1. Ma'ayan's experience reconfirmed my belief that healing is possible even after a horrendous birth experience.
2. There seems to be no limit to the resilience of a strong woman who is determined to reclaim her power and her health.
3. Ma'ayan achieved her vaginal birth without my presence in the delivery room. In my mind, that makes her story even more empowering.

Good Enough – Shlomit

Shlomit came to see me in her 41st week; she was after a myomectomy and a C-section. She was intent on birthing vaginally and couldn't find anywhere to do it. All the doctors she spoke with viewed her two uterine scars, and no one wanted to take a chance.

She had been in counseling with a colleague who referred Shlomit to me. She wanted to hear another opinion. Her story came right out of a book on posttraumatic maternity. Shlomit embodied so much of what I was learning and beginning to understand about women, trauma and birth.

She told the story backward, but I will tell it forwards. She was raised by two very strict parents. Her father beat her under the guise of proper parenting and discipline. She received very little love from either her mother or father. She suspected that she had a repressed history of sexual abuse, which had surfaced during a Rebirthing session. All through her childhood, she felt different from everyone else. She had a dreadful fear of authoritarian figures; she was terrified of men.

Shlomit is an athlete. She got involved in sports at a young age and eventually studied to be a physical education teacher. She used to play volleyball but turned elsewhere because it did not fulfill her need to challenge herself and prove what she was capable of achieving. She switched to the triathlon, a combination of long-distance running, swimming and biking. I was exhausted just hearing about it. When she talked about running on the beach, a smile spread across her entire face, and for the first time I could see her light.

Shlomit won first place in an Israeli triathlon competition. Her reaction to winning was that it probably was a mistake or that it was because the competition was substandard. She had trouble accepting her successes and achievements. Success didn't fit into her image of herself. Her father had instilled the belief that she would never be good enough and that whatever she did wasn't enough.

Three years before her first pregnancy, she had a large myoma which was removed by open uterine surgery. When she had the C-section, they removed the scar on her skin, but the scar remained on her uterus. In talking about myoma, she felt that it was the expression of all her frustrated and unexpressed emotions and her need to create something, to produce something tangible.

Three years later, she got pregnant. At 41 weeks she went to the clinic for a routine check-up. There was something suspicious on her monitor strip, and she was referred to the hospital. She went to one of the delivery rooms in Haifa. A young, inexperienced doctor freaked out when he estimated the baby's weight at five kilograms. He called in one of the senior consultants, and without even performing an additional weight estimation, they coerced her into agreeing to an elective C-section without a trial of labor. She explained that she had felt like a little girl when he talked to her. There was only one opinion – his. He reminded her of her father. She was unable to say or do anything. She was given no options. She was absolutely and completely speechless and helpless.

The C-section was a horrendous experience for her. She felt like a slab of meat. No one talked to her; no one even related to her in any manner. She didn't even remember that a midwife was present; she must not have made a big impression. The nurses tied her down to the table and immobilized both of her arms. She said that the only thing she could do was cry. At one point she escaped mentally because she couldn't stand being there anymore. It was more than she could handle. The baby weighed 3.900 kg.

In the recovery room, she asked the nurse to bring her the baby so she could breastfeed, which she successfully did. She was proud that she stood firm on the request, and she has fond memories of the nurse who was motherly, kind and patient with her.

Four years later she came to me in her 41st week, yearning for a natural birth. She was looking for control and to regain ownership of her body. She believed in her body and wanted to experience it doing its best work, bringing a baby into the world. She wanted to be like everyone else. She felt different and less worthy than other women. She felt that she was missing out on one of the most important things a woman can do in her life, give birth to her children.

She had not set a date for a repeat C-section. She went to Carmel Hospital in active labor; she had a quick first stage without any drugs but got stuck at full dilation. One of the senior doctors came into the room and asked her what she needed to push that baby out. She thought about it for a few moments and told him that she needed to stand up and feel the force of gravity. He invited her to do so, much to the surprise of the attending midwife. She brought the head to crowning by standing and leaning on the bed and climbed onto the bed just in time to push the baby out. This was an amazingly powerful experience for her. Her feeling of success was off the charts.

Lessons learned:

1. The thrill of an empowering birth experience lasts a very long time. I am still excited by this outcome. The thought of a woman creating a corrective birth experience for herself, especially after a C-section, is still exhilarating for me.
2. Help sometimes comes from unexpected sources. The senior physician's part in this story is significant and heart-warming. Shlomit managed to recruit him as an ally in her journey.
3. I believe that this work women do for themselves can and will change the world, one corrective birth experience at a time!
4. The secret to empowering women is to work with what is already there. Not every woman is a triathlon athlete, but every woman has strengths, internal resources and ways of coping with challenges. Sometimes she just needs someone to remind her how strong she is.

Finally Feeling the Urge

I first met Marian when she was in the 16th week of her second pregnancy. Her first birth culminated in a C-section at one of the hospitals in Haifa, and she was longing for a corrective experience. A friend of hers gave her my number. At our first meeting, the story of her first birth brought on an outpouring of tears and a whirlpool of disappointment, frustration, rage and hurt. She experienced feeling a loss of control.

Marian is an architect, but she was planning a career change in the direction of primary school education. She loves being in the company of children. Her husband Ephraim is an engineer. He is very intelligent and confident in his knowledge in the fields he has mastered. When he has to deal with areas of concern that he knows little or nothing about, he retreats and allows the experts to do their work. Marian is innately curious and instinctively seeks knowledge and mastery in all matters that cross her path.

Pregnancy and birth were no exception. Marian read books, participated in online discussion groups, did childbirth preparation and hired a doula to come with them to the hospital. After eight hours of active natural labor, she reached full dilation on her own steam. The midwife encouraged her to push, even though Marian didn't feel the urge at any point. She wanted to squat, but the midwife persuaded her to lie on her back instead of being upright. This was both confusing and frustrating for Marian and in direct conflict with everything she learned, knew and felt in her body.

The midwife didn't help her to get her baby out. Marian pushed on her back, while the midwife tugged on her perineum. After two-and-a-half hours, two doctors walked in and declared the need to operate. Her time was up. Marian refused. Then, a few minutes later, five doctors walked into the room, repeated the previous declaration and insisted that she consent to surgery. It was too much for her. She gave in.

Marian was dissatisfied with how the midwife had managed the second stage. She was disappointed that Ephraim had been so passive and reserved. She felt that he had put more trust in the doctors than in her. Marian resigned herself and signed the forms. In the operating room, before the surgery began, the baby's head was so low that the doctors asked the midwife to push the head up and out of the pelvis.

During the surgery, Marian disconnected herself from the proceedings. She even fell asleep at some point. The doctors and nurses were pleasant enough, but her attention was neither on their behavior nor their communication. They weren't interesting. Her major concern was the baby and when she could see him, touch him, hold him and breastfeed him. Nothing else was of any significance.

Postpartum, she compensated herself and baby Raphael for the bad birth by investing all her energy in full rooming-in and a good breastfeeding experience.

The second time Marian wanted a natural VBAC at Nazareth Hospital with me as her midwife. During our first meeting, she expressed interest in processing her negative birth experience, so we made an appointment to meet again a week later and started working together towards fashioning a plan for a healing and transformative birth experience.

Before we approached the topic of the birth, I wanted to assess her resources and get to know her better. I learned about the supportive and loving relationships she enjoys with her mother, father and brother. She is fortunate to be on the receiving end of unconditional love from her mother. Her relationship with her father combines mutual understanding and reciprocal intellectual stimulation. Her brother is one of her best friends.

She lives in a beautiful home that she and Ephraim own. As the result of an extensive renovation that she oversaw, their home is a beautiful, peaceful and serene refuge from the world. She is bright, analytical and sensitive, and she trusts herself. Her husband Ephraim is quiet, accepts and loves her as she is and provides her with feelings of inner strength, safety, stability and security.

When we first began discussing her birth, she wasn't able to call it a birth, because in her perception she didn't give birth. She used phrases like "They did this to me" and "This happened to me." I invited her to toy with the words, "I gave birth by Cesarean Section," but it didn't work for her. She saw the experience as passive because the baby had been pulled out of her; she had not given birth. She felt anger toward the midwife, and the very mention of her name brought up memories of her tugging on her perineum while urging her to push the baby out. The reaction of her body was disconnection and collapse.

The memory of the eight hours she spent successfully coping with natural labor until full dilation was almost inaccessible. I asked her to try and recall how the contractions felt, how she coped with them and how her body moved in reaction to them. We brought forth these memories and gave them time and space. Gradually she remembered what it was like to be in active labor, moving, breathing, and magnificently coping. She had a secure feeling in her back; her pelvis felt alive and relaxed.

From this place of connection to her strength, I asked Marian to look at the midwife again. She saw a young, sweet, inexperienced midwife who was not doing a very good job at getting this baby out. The anger Marian had been holding on to for over two years slipped away in a moment, and she felt a significant shift. The midwife transformed into a cartoonlike character who no longer triggered an emotional charge for Marian.

Our next major topic was Ephraim. Marian hadn't trusted him to support her during her first birth because he was so filled with fear. Even though her expectations were low, she was still disappointed. She doesn't trust him to support her now either. He tends to trust those in charge, not bothering to learn more or to get involved. He knows what he knows and doesn't know what he doesn't know. Marian is the opposite. She fights battles as they present themselves, sometimes not even pausing to check whether or not they are realistic. If she doesn't know something, she learns it. She cannot help but get involved.

I asked Marian to look around the clinic and choose two items to represent her and Ephraim. Marian chose two wooden figures from Africa, one female and one male. She experimented with their placement in relation to one another. She tried the male leading the female, in a protective position – that didn't work for her. She tried the female figure leading the way, with the male following behind – it felt better, but not precise. Standing side by side, sharing the way, deciding together felt even better. But, standing back-to-back, not agreeing, actually represented where they were at the time. She wanted a natural birth, and he wanted her to go for a repeat elective section. Ephraim and I needed to meet; I had to hear Ephraim's side of the story, because Marian wanted and needed him to be there by her side.

One week later I met Ephraim. He admitted that he has a lot of fears regarding doctors, hospitals and medical procedures. On the topic of birth, he chose to remain ignorant, and his lack of knowledge led him to experience a disabling loss of control during Marian's first birth. The obvious solution was for him to become knowledgeable, and he was willing and eager to begin learning. The next day he bought the book *Active Birth* and enthusiastically began reading. This is my all-time favorite book to recommend for those who want to start learning about the mechanisms of physiological birth from zero.

The next time we met, we started by using the knowledge Ephraim was acquiring to interpret what had happened during Marian's labor. We discovered a huge gap between how each of them had experienced the event. For Marian it was truly the end of the world, the worst-case scenario, the most awful thing that could happen. She expected Ephraim to speak up for her, be her voice and defend her position. He disappointed her terribly by not doing so, mostly because he was feeling relief and joy when they all made the decision to opt for surgery. For him, it was the best part of the birth. Marian burst into tears. We had hit rock bottom. The only direction from here was up. They would have a lot to talk about at home.

The next issue was touch. Marian considered Ephraim's touch to be "off" because he has weird, boney thumbs which he showed me. During the first birth, he was relieved of all expectations relating to touch, and the doula supported Marian physically. He was more of an observer and therefore felt like an outsider. I gave them homework, to explore the realm of touch, with Marian trying to be very explicit about what feels good and Ephraim trying everything and anything that she suggests. I encouraged them to become more comfortable with communicating by touching one another. They were excited about this.

They did their homework. Slowly Marian began to feel comfortable with Ephraim's touch. He also continued to read and become more and more knowledgeable. He was clearly on board and understood that his job involved being totally tuned in to Marian's needs, even when she did not verbalize them. Marian trusted him to do this because, from her experience, this is something he does well. They decided not to invite Marian's mother to be with them at the birth to make more room for Ephraim.

Marian was in and out of labor for a few days during weeks 39 and 40. She went past her due date, which was not an easy time for her. She had several false alarms during which she called in the troops. Ephraim came home from work which was an hour away, and her mother came to take care of Raphael. She went to Nazareth at precisely 41 weeks for a post-date check-up and unfortunately was met by some less-than-friendly doctors. She left crying and anxious. She received reflexology and shiatsu treatments; they helped her relax and center herself.

The labor started on Thursday night (41+2). Ephraim was at work, and she and Raphael were sleeping at her parents' house. The contractions started at about 10:30 pm. This time she knew it was the real thing because the contractions were painful. She waited to call both Ephraim and me just to make sure. I received a phone call at about midnight.

The contractions were six to seven minutes apart. Ephraim was still at work. We decided that she would call me when he got home unless something drastic happened, in which case she would ask her father to bring her to my place. I fell asleep until the next call and had a dream.

I dreamt that we were all together, and Marian was in active labor. She asked me to check her, and I debated whether to check her or myself. I decided to check myself and found a cervical dilation of six centimeters. We were both very happy and excited. I could feel the amniotic sac with my finger and played with it a bit. Then the cervix opened, and the baby started coming down so easily and smoothly that it was hard to believe. I asked Marian whether she wanted to give birth to the baby or whether she wanted me to do it, but it was too late to even decide because the baby was out and everything was good. I handed the baby to Marian; she held him to her chest and offered him a breast.

Then the phone rang, and it was Ephraim. I snapped myself out of the dream and reconnected to reality. Ephraim explained that he had just arrived home from work, had packed the car and they were on their way to my place. I popped into the shower, got dressed quickly, and ten minutes later they arrived. Marian was having contractions every three minutes; she was handling them well and was so happy and relieved to be in labor finally.

Ephraim looked a bit anxious but was also engaged and happy. He wanted us to get to the hospital ASAP, which was directly opposed to what Marian had planned. She wanted to get to the hospital as late as possible. Hearing the fetal heartbeat calmed him down a bit. Marian and I drank coffee, Ephraim drank tea, and pretty quickly it became obvious that Marian was in active labor.

She needed some support with breathing through the contractions, but her huge smile never left her face. She asked me to check her vaginally; she was five centimeters dilated. The dream suddenly reappeared in my consciousness. There was a curious but pleasant blurring of the boundaries between the real world and my dream world. I told Marian about the dream, and she laughed. She would have to birth this baby herself, and she was ready to do it.

Slowly we got organized and left together in the direction of the hospital in two cars. I called the delivery room in Nazareth from the road to let them know that we were coming. "Ahalaan wa'sahalaan habibti!" (Hello and welcome, my friend!) was the response.

We quickly arrived at the hospital; the entrance into the delivery room and the admitting process were both calm and quiet. We were more or less on our own. Marian got settled in with all her equipment, and soon after her waters broke. They were clear, the fetal monitor was perfect, the contractions were strong, Marian was excited and Ephraim was cautiously relaxed and present. Within less than two hours, she was fully dilated and feeling the urge to push.

The baby was born after less than a half-hour of spontaneous pushing. Ephraim held Marian's hand throughout the second stage and never let go. There were no lacerations, no cuts, no decelerations, no doctors and no drama. Marian was dazed and dumbfounded by how simple the whole process was. She took the baby to her chest and held him tightly. She repeated over and over, "I can't believe how much he looks like Raphael and how different he is from Raphael!" Different baby, different birth, different emotions, different sensations, same but different woman. She felt the baby come down, she felt the urge to push and she felt him find his way out. Only the last two contractions were painful.

From the point of view of having experienced a normal, physiological birth, Marian began to understand what had gone wrong the first time. Now, after experiencing the urge to push, she realized that she had been instructed to push for over two-and-a-half hours and never once actually felt a physical urge to push, even without an epidural.

She was able to let go of the anger, frustration and disappointment of her first birth. She now had her corrective experience. She wanted to take a shower and go home. Ephraim was happy, relieved and relaxed. He fully participated and witnessed the birth of his son and it was a wonderful experience for them as a couple.

When Marian saw how joyful he was, she declared that she is now ready to go forward with her plan to have five children.

Lessons learned:

1. Marian's journey was both empowering and healing. Ephraim also experienced something radically significant. They can barely remember how they were beforehand. Something shifted in their relationship and they became a different sort of couple; they were now much more of a team.
2. I am always thrilled to witness and act as a catalyst in the growth and development of young couples at the outset of their journey together.
3. In my mind, Marian is a sterling example of what can happen when a woman puts her healing at the center of her focus. She never looked back; her direction was always forward. She was dedicated to her purpose, and never let go. Two areas of growth stand out in my mind: her willingness to let go of the hurt and her unfaltering faith in Ephraim and their relationship. Everyone came out as winners.

VBAC, Hey!!!

I have known Alon since he was born and have been friends with his parents for over 40 years, since I moved to Israel. Alon was a happy, sweet and fun-loving child, who grew into a lovely young man. His wife Adva is an attorney. She is bright and sharp, and she knows what she wants. Adva and Alon came to me for help in achieving their dream, a vaginal birth after a Cesarean. We met several times, and they told me all about Adva's previous birthing experience.

The night before Adva's first birth, she felt contractions for several hours. Neither she nor Alon slept. She was 40+2 weeks. The next morning, she went to Rambam Hospital for a check-up. Her waters broke in the triage room. At first there were no real contractions and no dilation. Her progress was slow. Eventually she got to three cm., and with the help of Pitocin and an epidural, her cervix reached full dilation. She was told to push but felt nothing, and the baby's head didn't come down. After two and a half hours, the doctors told her she needed to be taken to the operating room for a Cesarean.

Before she signed the forms, she desperately tried to argue, to get explanations and get more time to ask questions. It didn't help. The situation was out of her control. Alon didn't join the argument. He just wanted to see the baby out and have the ordeal to be over. As a rule, he usually doesn't argue with people who know more than he does. Another part of him felt bad for Adva because he knew that this was exactly the opposite of what she wanted.

Alon managed to gain permission to be with her in the operating room, but when he came in, she was already unconscious. Apparently, they had given her some sedation. She had no memory of the operation. Alon experienced it as horrific. He was afraid that something terrible would happen to her. He couldn't take his eyes off the blood accumulating in the suction container.

When the baby was born, he felt nothing toward him other than anger for doing this to his wife. In the recovery room, Adva was afraid to close her eyes because she believed that she would die if she fell asleep. She kept herself alert by incessantly talking. She felt she might be going crazy.

In the postpartum ward, it took a while until she met her baby Ofek. In the meantime, she lashed out at Alon for not being on her side. She hadn't realized how much anger she had built up until it came out. Eventually, she started nursing the baby but had problems because of her inverted nipples. She got some help and slowly recovered from the surgery with the support of her family, friends, neighbors and a lactation consultant.

From early on, she knew that she would do everything in her power to ensure that her next birth would be different. She was not going to give her power away again.

On a warm April evening, I was just about to go to sleep when Adva called me at 11:30 pm to report that she was having regular contractions every eight minutes. She and Alon wanted to get organized, make sure their son Ofek was taken care of and then come over to the birth center.

According to the frequency of the contractions, it sounded a bit early, but there was something in Adva's voice that convinced me that this was the right thing to do. They needed to separate themselves from Ofek and focus on the birth. I told her that I trusted her instincts and that I was waiting for their arrival.

They left the house around midnight and reached the birth center at 12:30 am. When they arrived Adva was having contractions every five minutes, and she was managing them well. Fifteen minutes later, while she was sitting on my beige and white couch, her waters suddenly broke. She managed to jump up before any damage was done. We tried to find a way for her to be comfortable with amniotic fluid dripping out of her with each contraction.

She found a rhythm by breathing, swaying and being touched and held by Alon. The contractions became stronger and much closer together, and at 1:45 I examined her. She was five centimeters dilated. This was really good news. We decided to get ready to drive to Carmel Hospital where she planned on having her VBAC. She decided on Carmel because she had heard they have the highest successful VBAC rate in the North. I called ahead to let them know that we were on our way.

We drove in two cars. It was a foggy night, and the road was empty. There was plenty of parking near the hospital, and we slowly made our way to the delivery room. It was temporarily located in the basement of the hospital during a two-and-a-half-year-long renovation. They took us straight into a delivery room, circumventing triage.

Two of the three midwives on duty were very quiet and disinterested. Maybe they were just tired. The third was friendly and welcoming. We did not get the friendly one, but she did come in to say hello and check on Adva several times. Each time she came in, Adva begged her to stay with us, but she mumbled something incomprehensible and apologetically left the room.

Adva was hooked up to a fetal monitor and told that it would be for about half an hour. She ended up attached to that monitor continuously for close to ten hours. Adva asked each midwife and doctor who came into the room when she could go off the monitor, go to the toilet and take a shower. No one said either yes or no; no one explained whether the monitor was normal or not. Again, something incomprehensible was mumbled to her, and she remained attached to the monitor. The fetal heartbeat had good variability and went down slightly during each contraction but remained within the range of normal at all times.

It was nearly impossible for Adva to find a comfortable position in bed. An IV line was put in, blood was taken and she was given antibiotics because she was GBS positive. At around 4 am, after she was examined by the OB, Adva had a three-minute-long contraction, which was followed by another series of strong contractions. The fetal heartbeat went down to

80-100 bpms and didn't recover completely. The doctor had stripped her membranes without asking for consent or explaining his actions.

A senior resident was called in, and he gave orders for IV Atosiban, amnioinfusion, IUP and fetal scalp electrode. Within minutes, the birth took on an atmosphere of an intensive care case. Adva was asked to remove her jewelry and sign a consent form for a C-section. I checked to see if Alon was OK. He was worried about the baby but was present and engaged.

The baby's heart rate beat recovered, and Adva went back to trying to manage the contractions. She had two instruments sticking out of her vagina, one attached to the baby's scalp and the other in her uterus. She was wet, tired and in pain. There was a cervical dilation of eight centimeters. She couldn't get comfortable, and not long afterward, at about 5:30, she asked for an epidural.

At about 6:00 am daylight entered the room from the high windows. With the help of the epidural, Adva rested from the pain of the contractions, and Alon fell asleep on the lounger. At 6:40 her cervical dilation was nine centimeters, but the head was still high. Our thoughts swung back and forth between hope for a vaginal birth and the real possibility of a repeat cesarean section. The head was high and the fetal monitor was less than perfect. Adva never lost hope, not for a split second. She provided enough inspiration for all of us to remain optimistic.

About a half-hour later more light entered the room, but this time it was in human form. A midwife named Anat joined us for her morning shift and brought with her a glow of confidence and compassion that lit up the room. Adva fell in love with her instantly. Anat was young, pretty, smart, gentle and laid back. I knew her because she had been with me at a home birth as a student midwife. More importantly, she had confidence in Adva's ability to give birth.

She shared her thoughts, and together we made a plan. The administration of antibiotics would need to continue because Adva was GBS positive and her membranes were ruptured for a long time.

She would need to be catheterized so that a full bladder would not impede the progress of the baby's head. Anat promised to get rid of all the wet sheets and get some clean ones. Anat and I would get her into an upright position to encourage the head to go down. At 8:00 Adva was fully dilated, but the head was still high.

I got busy working with Adva with the aid of the birth ball. She laid on her side with one leg on the ball; we did hip circles, rocking in all directions, in an attempt to create as much movement as possible in her pelvis and to allow the baby's head to come down. At 9:45 the head had come down to S+1, and Anat began working with Adva to see if she could push the baby down and out. Every effort she made brought the head down a little bit more, and with every effort, there was a slight deceleration in the baby's heartbeat followed by a full recuperation. This was a fetal monitor for believers in babies' capacity to endure birth.

Unfortunately, a major nonbeliever appeared suddenly in the room, Dr. A. She didn't like the fetal monitor; she didn't believe that Adva would give birth vaginally. She started hinting that she wanted this baby out, preferably with help of knives and other instruments.

A battle began between optimism and pessimism, a medical approach to birth and a holistic midwifery approach, light and dark, good and evil. Anat negotiated these two worlds with the elegance of a veteran. She had danced this dance many times before. She assured us that everything would be okay and that Adva would succeed in giving birth vaginally. We believed her. All the signs indicated that she was right, and if we could just keep the doctor out of the room long enough, there was a chance that it could actually happen.

At about 10:45 we began to see the head during the contractions in response to Adva's almost superhuman efforts to push this baby out. Dr. A. wasn't convinced. She was more impressed by the non-reassuring monitor and the head's tendency to rise back into the pelvis in between contractions. Both of these are typical for a birth in which the umbilical cord is wrapped around the baby's neck. In between contractions the fetal heartbeat was reassuring, and we were all reassured, except Dr. A.

She wanted this birth transferred to the operating room just in case there would be the need for an intervention. She presented her case to all of us, and there was no room for an argument. After she left the room, Anat turned to Adva and told her not to worry, that there will be no interventions. She recommended that she ignore everything that was going on around her and just keep pushing. In the worst-case scenario, the baby would be born in the operating room.

And that was exactly what happened. We moved like an entire circus caravan in the elevator down to the operating room, which included: Adva (pushing), Alon (a bit in shock), two young residents (following orders), Anat (conducting the orchestra), me (having flashbacks of similar absurd situations during my hospital days) and the orderly who transported Adva in the bed, together with a fetal monitor, an incubator and the vacuum machine. Wouldn't it have been easier to just stay in the delivery room? The head was on the perineum, and no one would dare operate on Adva at this stage anyway. Dr. A. wasn't even a part of the convoy; she had remained in the delivery room to hold down the fort.

There was another flash of warm light and some really good news when we arrived in the operating room. The Ob/Gyn waiting for us was the head of the department, a doctor who is known for his patience and for his belief in women's ability to give birth. Alon and I weren't present because we weren't allowed in. We were told later by Anat that he took one look at the monitor, lifted the sheet, saw the baby's head halfway out and didn't understand what all the fuss was about. After two contractions the baby was born, and Adva was glowing in the light of her victory. Anat took pictures and captured the moment. Adva did it. VBAC HEY!

The umbilical cord was wrapped around the baby's neck, but she was born full of vigor, luminosity and vitality. She was ready to meet her beautiful, brave mother, her sweet, loving father and her charming, curious brother Ofek. It was quite a dramatic entry into the world!

Lessons learned:

1. When the umbilical cord is wrapped around the baby's neck, the fetal monitor can be pretty scary, the progress may be slow and the head will come down only at the very last minute. This is a birth that requires belief both in the mother and the baby. An optimistic midwife who believes that everything will be okay does so based on knowledge and experience.
2. Adva's strong motivation to succeed affected the outcome of this birth. Her dedication to her goal brought out the superhuman powers within her.
3. It inspires me over and over to connect with birth professionals who are knowledgeable, confident and kind. There are islands of sensibility within what seems like an ocean of fear, politics, personal interests, ego struggles and defensive medicine. There are so many good people doing this work.

Noa's Cesarean Party

There are things I know because I am a human being with a healthy brain, a good heart and a strong body. There are things I know because I am a woman and a mother who has given birth, raised three children and become a grandmother. There are things I know because I have been working as a midwife for twenty-seven years and have witnessed and participated in many births. Over the years, I have acquired a new type of knowledge, that of a trauma therapist. I have heard the difficult stories of many very disturbing births. With Noa, I had a rare opportunity to tie together all these different threads of knowledge and participate in a corrective birth experience that took place in the operating room of Nazareth Hospital.

Noa came to me during the 36th week of her second pregnancy. Her first birth had culminated in an emergency C-section due to the failure of the baby to make progress in its descent through the birth canal. As an experienced midwife, it saddened me to realize that I didn't hear anything really out of the ordinary in Noa's story. She was induced at 41 weeks due to a reduced amount of amniotic fluid. She spent several days in the delivery room with neither food nor drink. She received an early epidural due to her exhaustion and the loss of her ability to cope with her contractions. An internal fetal monitor and amnioinfusion were inserted, and after three hours of directed pushing, she was taken to a C-section.

As a woman and a mother, this sounds like a long, distressing and frightening story. As a midwife, I also worry about the baby. Where is she in this story? She was also in labor all those hours. What was the fetal outcome? I pray that they both are okay. As a human being, I also think of her spouse, Amnon, and his place in this scenario.
How did he manage during all those hours? I hope that someone cared for him, supported him, and brought him sandwiches and coffee. I also wonder about Noa, lying in bed for all those hours without going crazy. How could anyone stay sane without eating for so long?

Wasn't she starving? How did she find the strength to go on?

In the clinic, as a body-mind psychotherapist, I sat with Noa and listened to her story, as her inner experience unraveled. We sat together, slowed down the pace of time, paid attention to every detail of the incident and began to understand what happened to her there. What emotions did she feel, what thoughts went through her mind and what sensations did she experience in her body? By pinpointing what went wrong and recognizing her needs for her upcoming birth, Noa planted the seeds for a corrective experience.

We started from the beginning. From the moment the decision was made to perform the C-section, there was a drastic and unexpected increase in the number of actions performed by multiple caregivers all at the same time. This put Noa into a whirlwind of confusion, helplessness and loss of control. She lost her ability to absorb, understand and cooperate. She felt like an object, not a person.

She had a clear memory of the dry shaving of her pubic hair without any soap and water and feeling sore. She also had a strange and clear memory of various objects being placed on her body while she was being prepared for surgery in the delivery room. She remembers thoughts going through her head like, "Am I actually being used as a shelf? A table? Is this even real?"

Her transfer to the operating room was frightening and fast. She lost Amnon somewhere along the way and didn't get to properly say goodbye with a hug and a kiss. She found herself alone in a frozen room full of instruments, machines and strangers wearing robes, masks and hats. No one approached her; no one talked to her. Someone took her eyeglasses, so she couldn't see well. This increased her sense of disorientation, confusion and helplessness. And it was really cold! The cold penetrated her bones; she was already trembling with fear. It was impossible to differentiate between the two.

The scrubbing of her naked belly and legs with soap and water before the surgery intensified the sensation of cold, and together with the experience of exposure, it created a very difficult moment for Noa. She was alone, trembling, exposed, helpless, unable to see and with no one to talk to and nowhere to escape.

During the operation, the nurses and doctors talked among themselves on subjects unrelated to the surgery. She felt her organs being moved around like pieces of meat. The feeling wasn't pleasant, but she realized that it was something she had to suffer. Her focus was elsewhere. She was waiting to hear crying, waiting to meet her baby, waiting to hear that everything is fine and waiting for this to all end.

She is told that the baby is out. She hears crying but doesn't see her. A green sheet serving as a vertical divider between her head and the rest of her body blocks her view. Noa is told that her baby girl is being taken care of by the midwife. Her body cries out. She yearns to see her, feel her, hold her in her arms, hug her and smell her. The midwife approaches her with a green bundle, and she brings it closer to her. Through blurry vision, she sees a sweet face and bursts into tears. Her tears are a mishmash of joy, relief, excitement, loss, fear, disappointment and love.

The midwife brings the baby's cheek to hers. She cries into Noa's ear. She wants to hold her baby but can't because both of her arms are tied down. The desire to hold her baby turns into the need to hold her and then into anger and frustration. Her hands are weeping. She thinks to herself "For what purpose do I have hands if not for cradling my baby when she cries?"

The midwife goes away and takes Noa's precious green package with her. The pediatrician is waiting. They prepare to take the baby to the newborn unit to warm her. The door closes behind them, and there is silence. She is alone again in the cold with the strangers, the smell of her blood, the feeling of raw and exposed flesh and her tethered hands. It feels like an eternity. She thinks to herself: "Did I give birth? This doesn't feel how birth should feel."

She is moved into recovery. Alone again. Her body is still shaking with cold, excitement and shock. There are new blurry faces. She thinks for a moment that her husband must be together with the baby in the newborn unit. It's a little reassuring but also fills her with envy. She says to herself, "After giving birth, a baby should be with his mother, right?" Nothing happened according to the plan. Noa is exhausted, sore and trembling. A nurse places a warm blanket on Noa's shaking body, and she is comforted by the warmth.

Amnon comes into the recovery room with a smile from ear to ear. He is a happy man. He is a father. He has a baby girl! He tells her how the whole family has arrived, and everyone has already seen the baby. He shows her pictures on his mobile phone in which he is holding the baby, her grandmother is holding her and the nurse in the ward is taking care of her.

She is so beautiful, but Noa only feels a cold stone in her heart, and she thinks, "Everyone has held her except me." She didn't want a baby whom everyone has already touched, just like a mother cat who doesn't want a kitten that strangers have touched. It took her a long time for Noa to build a healthy connection with her daughter after this traumatic beginning.

There is more to tell, but I choose to stop here because I want to write about the healing process.

Noa and Amnon asked me to accompany them to their birth in the delivery room. Noa decided that she wanted to aim for a natural birth this time but not at all costs. We continued to meet, and together we created a birth plan. This time Noa hoped to experience control, sharing, empowerment, respect, calm, marital intimacy and an immediate connection with the baby.

During week 41, at a postdate check-up at the hospital, a deceleration was spotted on the fetal monitor, and Noa was immediately admitted to the delivery room. I drove to Nazareth to be with them. My first act was to play some soothing music, and then the three of us talked quietly. Noa realized that there were two options: surgery now or surgery later. She decided on surgery now. I left the room to allow the two of them to continue to process their decision, cry a little, breathe a little and digest the turn of events.

I inform the doctor of their decision and begin to collect equipment in preparation for the surgery. I recall the excessive speed with which the previous preparation was done, and consciously make sure I do things differently this time. I knock on the door, wait for permission to enter and find Noa crying. She calms me down by explaining that these are tears of excitement in anticipation of meeting her son.

We start with the shave. Noa asks to take a shower before the surgery. She also asks for an enema. After creating a plan together, I shave Noa with warm water and soap and administer the enema. She uses the toilet and takes a shower and returns after ten minutes, emptied, squeaky clean and ready to go.

A female doctor comes in to take blood tests and insert the IV line. There's a discussion about the site of the insertion of the needle. Noa doesn't want it on her wrist because according to her experience, it hurts too much there. The doctor cooperates, and together they find a place that is acceptable to both. She signs the consent form for the surgery. The doctor writes orders for premedication. Everything is done slowly. Noa asks questions and gets answers. She removes her jewelry and gives it to Amnon for safe keeping. She does not take off her glasses; this time she wants to see.

Noa moves over to the stretcher. We all go together in the elevator. It is crowded and cozy. Everyone is smiling and taking pictures. We all go into the operating room together. An anesthesiologist and an operating room nurse approach us; this is standard procedure in preparation for surgery. There are questions, and there are answers.

Noa has some requests. She would like to keep her glasses on so she can see her baby, and she would like to have one arm free so she can hold him. There are some grimaces, glances are exchanged, eyebrows are raised, there is some tension and finally there is an answer, "Yes, why not?" There is a short discussion between the anesthesiologist and the OR nurse regarding the glasses, and in the end, there is a decision, a compromise. As long as the diathermy is working, no glasses.

When her baby is out, her glasses will be put in place so that she can see him. There is a lovely feeling of collaboration. Noa has a feeling of control and appreciates the consideration of her needs. I count the small victories, one at a time.

Noa enters the operating room with me by her side. It is really cold. I stand by her, offering explanations and distractions while the spinal block is performed and she is prepped for surgery. The mood is good, everyone seems calm. The doctors are working slowly and carefully. I prepare Noa for the moment when she will hear her baby's cry, and that's what happens. I put her glasses in place, and the anesthesiologist releases her arm from the restraint. The midwife brings Noa's baby to her, and she holds, hugs, kisses, feels, smells and sees her sweet son. Photographs are taken. Many tears of joy are shed.

The anesthetist asks Noa if she wants to sleep while her belly is being closed up, and she answers him that yes, she will gladly go to sleep. I decide to stay; I don't want anything to spoil the magic. I don't want her to open her eyes and discover that she is alone. I sit, rest, breathe and notice how much happiness there is in my heart. This was truly a Cesarean Party.

I wait for the surgery to end. I thank everyone graciously and accompany Noa to the recovery room. Amnon informs us of the baby's weight with a text message. All is well; no one is alone. I'm with Noa and Amnon is with the baby. Later, Amnon comes into the recovery room. A curtain is closed around us, and we are asked to be quiet. I decide to go and leave Noa and Amnon alone, together. I tell them that I'll meet them upstairs.

Immediately upon her arrival in the maternity ward, Noa requests that they bring her baby to breastfeed, and she is brought in immediately. We peel off all the fabrics in which she is wrapped because Noa wants to feel her naked skin on hers. I cover both of them with warm blankets, and the baby makes her way to the breast and latches on. I can feel my breath calm down just a little bit more.

I say my goodbyes. None of us was able to find the words to express the enormity of what we had just experienced together, so we left things unspoken. There were many hugs.

Lessons learned:

1. All the types of my knowledge came together uniquely during this birth. I felt a special cooperation between the person in me, the woman in me, the midwife in me and the therapist in me which allowed something amazing to happen.
2. Things can always be better. The cooperation of the nurses and doctors was especially moving for me. They worked differently that day. They put the patient in the center and their personal convenience and the protocols aside. I got the impression that this was also an empowering experience for them. We met their humanity and not the uniforms or masks that they often hide behind.
3. This story touched many women. I published it on my Facebook page, and the responses were overwhelming. In retrospect, I contemplate that maybe that day we invented the concept of the mother-and-baby-friendly C-section.

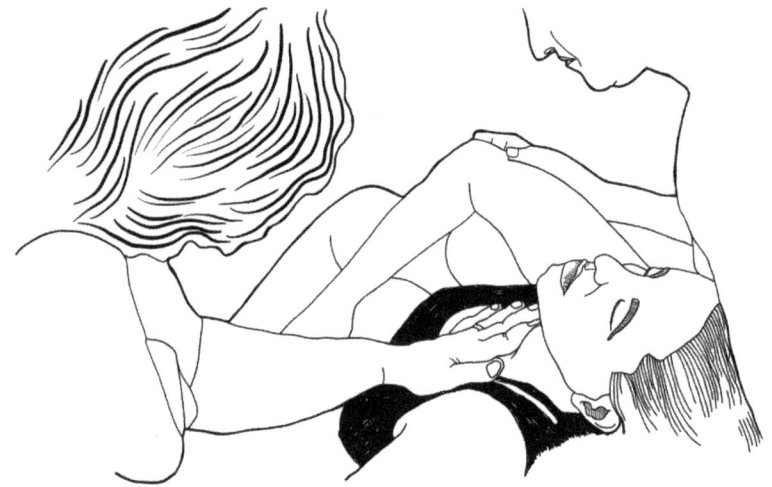

Inspiring Work with Abuse Survivors

Throughout the years, I have worked with at least 100 survivors of sexual violence. Some of them suffered childhood sexual abuse, some were rape victims and some were both. At first my work was mostly instinctual and midwifery based. I focused on empowering these women and helping them to get back their sense of control. They planned their births meticulously, trying to anticipate the pitfalls. Gradually as I read, studied, trained, met more women and gained more experience, my focus shifted. The body became the locus of attention. This shift was the key to enabling healing to manifest through the birth experience. I am so grateful to the women who taught me everything I know about this special corner of the world. They were my teachers and my guides through the maze of post-trauma and its winding paths of pain, courage, discovery and the warm light of healing.

The Births of Aya and Noga

Tali and Uri called me early in Tali's pregnancy, during her seventh week. When we met face to face, she was in her ninth week. She became the first member of a select group of women who entered my life immediately after their pregnancy tests showed positive. These women gently but firmly brought me into a new realm of midwifery. I began doing true, responsible, evidence-based, holistic and professional prenatal care. Finally, I felt like a real midwife. I buried myself in the midwifery textbooks and relearned what I had forgotten, this time highlighting the practical aspects.

Tali had already been pregnant three times; she had been through two miscarriages and an abortion. She and Uri were both very happy about the current pregnancy and the new baby, especially Uri, who seemed to be the more emotional member of this couple. Tali was more cautious with expressing her feelings, especially to newcomers in her life. She made it clear from the beginning that it would take time for her to let me in, and one thing we certainly had at our disposal was time.

Uri is a chef, organic nutritionist, cooking teacher and foodie. He researches the history of food and nutrition in the Middle East and has startling amounts of knowledge on the topic. Every visit to their house included a delicious and creative breakfast made by Uri. He exposed me to foods, tastes and aromas I didn't even know existed.

Tali was set on having a home birth. She had researched it extensively through books and the internet, and she had vast amounts of knowledge about pregnancy, birth and mothering. She not only read but also retained knowledge and remembered what she had researched. Our conversations were always stimulating and thought-provoking.

As a child, Tali suffered from a problem with her nose, and she underwent surgery eight times. As a result, she developed a strong distaste and distrust for doctors and hospitals. She also suffered from gallstones and treated herself with herbal remedies and nutrition.

In addition, she was in a bus accident and suffered a strong blow to her head. During our second meeting, she also told me about her childhood experiences of sexual abuse. I told her about my thesis and my interest in trauma and birth. We both felt that we had discovered a solid basis for a good connection.

Throughout the pregnancy, we got to know each other very, very gradually. Tali is a private person in many ways. She doesn't share her emotions or her body easily with those around her. Explicit consent was necessary for a hug or a pat on her pregnant belly. Building trust was a process that took time. Nothing was assumed. Every word and every action had to be tested, discussed and either accepted or rejected. At times I felt like I was walking on eggshells.

Even though being with her wasn't easy, I learned to like and respect her a lot. She forced me to push myself beyond my comfort zone in many realms of my midwifery, and she taught me new ways of thinking by questioning accepted practices. Her mind was constantly working; each time we met, she brought up a new topic that compelled us to create solutions that fit both her and my approaches. It was a sort of intellectual wrestling match in which we both fought to come out together on top, holding hands in consensus.

Tali and Uri made an interesting request that I had never encountered before. They asked me to meet with both sets of parents to calm them down and convince them that I was a serious, safe and experienced midwife. No pressure. It was actually fun in the end. The grandparents were curious, sweet, excited and a little bit worried. I understood their concerns, legitimized them and answered all of their questions. I think the meeting went well. Before we parted, I gave them my phone number and assured them that they could call me if they needed to ask any more questions or voice any more concerns.

At first, Tali and Uri had considered birthing alone without a midwife, but they were afraid to take all the responsibility upon themselves. They compromised by hiring me, and they made it very clear that they wanted to do as much as possible by themselves, both during the pregnancy and during the birth.

Regarding her pregnancy follow-up, Tali agreed to do one organ scan and agreed to listen to the baby's heart tones only with the Pinard fetoscope. During the birth, she did not want to be examined, and she did not want to hear the baby's heart tones more than was necessary. She wanted to be alone with Uri as much as possible, and she wanted my presence to not be felt at all.

I took none of this personally. I understood completely that it was coming from her difficulty trusting people. There was a lot of unspoken understanding between us even though Tali chose not to directly address her abuse issues. We talked around them and dealt with specific requests as they surfaced during the pregnancy.

One issue that became central as the birth approached was her lack of willingness and/or readiness to accept help. As the birth became imminent, she expressed more and more apprehension regarding help, touch and contact. I began to wonder how I was going to do my job without touching, helping and being in intimate contact. This is how I do my job. These are the tools that I have perfected throughout the years. This is what I do best.

As the birth approached, I started losing sleep, wondering how things would turn out. I tried to imagine myself invisible and silent. It did not put me at ease. I can be quiet, but I'd never done "invisible" before. Deep in my heart, I knew that Tali was silently crying out for affection, contact and support, but she couldn't find the way to recognize, come to terms with or verbalize these needs. I was hoping that the birth would provide an opening for her that would help her to recognize the rewards of being loved and cared for.

On March 11, Shabbat, I received a phone call from Uri at 1 pm, in which he informed me that Tali had been having contractions since 4 am, and during the last half hour they were coming every five minutes. He reported that Tali was coping easily with the pain using positions, breathing and relaxation techniques. He was in charge of food and drinks. They sounded just fine. At 4 pm the contractions were coming every three minutes and were becoming more painful. They asked me to come to their home. I took a deep breath, got my equipment together and drove to Kfar Yehoshua.

I found Tali in the living room standing and hanging from a metal bar that ran parallel to the ceiling. She paced and chatted during the breaks, but as the pain mounted, she became quiet, closed her eyes and breathed silently with her arms stretched over her head. When the contraction passed, she slowly returned her consciousness to our world and chit-chatted hesitantly. I could feel that my presence was uncomfortable for her. I followed her lead and did no more or no less than she did or asked for. I was quiet during the contractions and talked and joked quietly with her during the breaks.

Slowly the intensity of the contractions accelerated; they were coming every three minutes and were over a minute long. The chatting ended and Tali started to channel all her energy into coping with the contractions and resting during the breaks. I could see on her face that the level of her pain was mounting. I listened to the baby's heartbeat and suggested a warm shower.

The shower helped, but after its soothing effects passed, Tali searched for another source of relief and she couldn't find one on her own. I suggested a glass of wine. Wine has a way of calming women in labor, allowing their bodies to take over and reset the system. The effect of the alcohol can go one of two ways, either by enabling a short, needed rest (or even sleep) or by lowering inhibitions and allowing the birth to intensify and move forward. Tali agreed to a glass of red wine.

After the wine, I suggested a massage. I didn't know exactly who would be massaging her, but it seemed like a good idea when the words came out of my mouth. Blurting out this suggestion was my first real spontaneous action at this birth; maybe it was the wine. There was a short, awkward pause between my words and Tali's response.

She responded that yes, she would love a massage and that Uri is no good at it at all. She agreed that I would be the one.

Before she could retract from her moment of willingness, I grabbed my oils and encouraged her to find a comfortable position. Leaning forward and still in her bathrobe, she and Uri created a mound of pillows into which she burrowed her body and found a good spot. I poured aromatic oil on both of my hands and began massaging her lower back, her shoulders and her neck, gradually progressing to her buttocks, legs and arms. We were all silent. The only sound I could hear was our breathing and the sliding of my hands moving over her body. She whimpered through the first few contractions and then became very still, and fell asleep.

At 7:35 pm, Tali woke up suddenly with a very strong contraction and a cry of surprise and delight as her waters broke. The contractions were back and were coming every three minutes. Things were moving in the right direction; the wine had done its magic. Tali got comfortable sitting on the birthing stool. I had a feeling she would like the modesty it affords and she did.

Uri sat in front of her, I sat beside her and we held her, massaged her back, and breathed together with her through the contractions. All awkwardness was gone, we were working together and Tali was doing it. The contractions were much more painful than she had anticipated; she was having a hard time. Uri and I saw an amazing woman doing an amazing job. She felt out of control and beyond her ability to cope. Pushing two clenched fists into Uri's chest was one way she found to get through the contractions. At 11:30 pm she asked me to examine her and we discovered a dilation of eight centimeters, 100% effacement, and the head at S–2.

At about midnight she started feeling a little pressure. I knew that she wanted to avoid pushing until the very last minute, so I suggested that she get into bed and lie down on her side. She was tired and feeling kind of woozy and spaced out, so the idea of lying down was a good one for many reasons. She rested in between contractions, cursed and breathed through the contractions. She was in the transition phase. At about 1:10 she started pushing very gently on her side. I phoned Maya soon after and asked her to join us.

Maya arrived at about 2 am, and I could see the head pressing on Tali's perineum from within. I suggested that we move over to the birthing stool and get set up for the birth. Tali felt good on the stool. She was comfortable; it felt familiar to her and she could maintain her modesty. No one was peering at her perineum while watching her push her baby out. It was all happening under the chair.

Aya was born at 2:30. She took a little while to come around, but I could tell that she was with us from the beginning. She was beautiful and landed in her mother's arms, where she stayed for a long, long time! Her breathing was a little noisy and she snored a bit, but her color was fine and she looked happy.

Uri was ecstatic. Tali seemed to be a bit shell-shocked; she didn't quite believe that she had survived this ordeal. I could barely believe it myself, that I had survived this entire pregnancy and seen the birth to its fruition. Everything was just fine. We were all fine.

I sent Maya home after the placenta came out. There was a small tear that didn't warrant suturing. Tali got settled in with Aya in bed, propped up on a big pile of pillows. They looked into each other's eyes, getting used to the idea of each other's existence. Uri took lots of pictures of the new reality and made phone calls to all the new grandparents, aunts and uncles. There was a collective sigh of relief.

A few days later, Tali and I talked about the birth. She was overwhelmed by the pain and the intensity of the whole experience. She felt out of control and disappointed in herself for not being able to cope in the manner she had anticipated. I saw things differently. I saw a woman opening up, giving birth to her daughter and giving birth to a new self. I saw a woman who discovered that help is a good thing, that support comes in many forms, that new people can be trusted and that her body is a source of power and strength.

She remembered very clearly the experience of the massage and of falling asleep. It was a turning point for both of us. It was when I became myself and allowed my skills and experience to come forward. It was when Tali allowed herself to just "be" when she let go of the control that she thought would get her through the birth and when she let her body take over. I believe that her birth was a healing experience. It would take some time for her to see it. She was still lost in the fog of the intensity.

About a year later, Uri called and I understood immediately that Tali was pregnant again. They wanted me to be their midwife again. Another rollercoaster ride, another egg walk and another learning experience. Tali has a way of teaching me lessons that come from the least expected places. This turned out to be even truer this time than the last.

Our first meeting was on Pesach, the morning after the Seder. It was an odd time to be working, but that was their request. I had no reason to object because I had nothing special planned. Tali poured her heart out at that meeting. She told me how difficult her first birth had been for her. She had suffered physically, mentally, emotionally and spiritually. She was disappointed in herself, angry at the birth world for not telling her the truth about how painful birth is and, more than anything, she was scared to death to go through it again. Her wish was to go to sleep and wake up with a baby in her arms. She also made it clear that she wanted to feel my presence even less this time than last. She asked me to stay in the garden as much as possible.

The pregnancy was uneventful except for its length. She went to 42+4 (or over 43, depending on who's counting). At 42 weeks, she and Uri went to the Nazareth Hospital for an ultrasound and monitor. Everything was normal, so we went forward into the uncharted territory of the 43rd week. I went through different phases during the days we spent in that 43rd week: phases of fear, hope, faith and sheer terror (stillbirth, thick meconium, big baby, post-term syndrome). I asked her to go to the hospital again in the middle of the week. She planned to go to the hospital the morning she went into labor.

Tali's contractions started during the night. As the morning approached, they got longer and closer together. I spoke with Uri on the phone twice. He reported that Tali was doing fine and that Aya was with Tali's sister at the neighbor's house. The phones were disconnected, and they were as disengaged from the world as they could possibly be, living in the middle of a very active organic vegetable farm. Uri told me that he was doing some last-minute food shopping for the meals that Tali had asked him to prepare for the birth.

I knew she would not agree to go to the hospital with contractions, so I didn't even suggest that she get checked out before active labor kicked in. What I did raise was the volume on my faith dial and got ready to go to their house. I stopped on the way and bought a book. Until I learned to knit, reading would have to make do as an adequate substitute. I planned to pass the time in the garden with my new book.

I arrived at about 12:30 to the pungent aroma of goulash cooking on the stove. I found Tali in Uri's office surrounded by books and computers. It seemed to me to be an odd place to labor, among the machines, but the reasoning behind it was that Tali was watching a movie on the laptop to keep her mind occupied during the breaks. During the contractions, Uri rubbed her back, held her tightly and told her over and over how much he loved her, how strong she is, and how he is there for her. She leaned her head on a water bottle on Uri's desk and got through the contractions one by one. I listened to the baby's heartbeat, and it sounded fine. We discussed how far away they wanted me to be, and Tali's response was as far as possible. As far as she was concerned, I could go home. Uri wanted me closer. I went outside and looked for a place to locate myself.

I left the Doppler with Uri, settled into a hammock in the garden and started reading my book. It was a beautiful day. I almost fell asleep. After about an hour I knocked on the door, let myself in and found that things seemed to be progressing nicely. The contractions were getting longer, Tali was making labor sounds and Uri was happy.

He had listened to the baby's heartbeat and reported to me that everything was fine. I didn't tell him, but I had been listening through the door and heard for myself. Uri served me some goulash, and I settled into a rocking chair in the living room. I listened to Tali's reactions to her contractions as they gradually strengthened. She maintained her sense of humor. She freely expressed her reactions to the pain, alternating with her frustration concerning the way babies are brought into the world. I listened to the baby's heartbeat again and went outside.

Outside I walked around a bit, made some phone calls and read some more. There was a lot of activity on the farm, but Tali was completely oblivious to it. There was construction going on right under her window, cars coming in and out and farm workers going about their day. No one seemed to be aware of the fact that a baby was coming into the world, that a woman was suffering so much pain in order to let it happen, that her husband was doing everything and anything possible to do and say the right things at the right times and that I was walking around, wondering what my part was in all this and how to be present without violating Tali's space.

I went inside again and found Tali in much more intense labor. It seemed that every time I left and came back, her labor seemed to progress. She cried, she shouted, she punched Uri a bit here and there. She expressed exactly what she was feeling, and the range of emotions was enormous. She laughed at herself and cried a lot. She showered until the hot water ran out and wondered how she would manage without it.

The house was getting cold, and I asked Uri to light the wood stove. He was happy to do so. After hearing the baby's reassuring heartbeat again, I went to the neighbors' house for a cup of coffee; we all sat around the kitchen table and chatted. Their house was so warm that the fan was on. I noticed the contrast in temperatures between the two neighboring houses. It seemed odd.

At about 4 pm I went back to the house, to Tali. The house was warm, and the smell of burning wood was in the air. Her contractions were becoming very painful. She was suffering and considered filling the birth pool. I suggested a vaginal check in order to avoid getting busy with the pool if the birth seemed imminent. She was nine centimeters dilated. Great!

At 4:40 I called Sarahle and asked her to come to join us. I started getting ready for the baby's arrival. I prepared my equipment, gathered what Tali had prepared and set up the birth chair in front of the wood-burning stove. She was in the shower, and the hot water ran out again. She was frantic again about how she would manage without the comfort it provided. She came into the living room in her bathrobe.

She tried sitting on the birth chair, but it didn't feel right. She found herself on all fours on the mattress in the corner. The contractions were very strong, and she had trouble finding a comfortable position. I offered her the birth ball which was good for only a few contractions.

Sarahle arrived; I went outside to talk to her in the car for a minute. Tali requested that she remain in the car unless she was needed. That was not a problem for Sarahle. When I came back into the house, I found Tali on all fours ON TOP of Uri, who was also on all fours. She tried pushing gently, but it hurt. I told her to stop. Obviously, there was still a cervical lip. Pushing should not hurt.

I massaged her back through her terry cloth bathrobe. No words were spoken, and gradually she relaxed and calmed down a bit. The urge to push reappeared. This time there was no pain and apparently, the lip was gone. She started pushing, groaning and grunting with each contraction. They were coming approximately every four minutes. Tali rested during the breaks, sprawled over Uri's back. When asked, he said that he was OK, but he was very relieved when suddenly Tali decided that she wanted to get up and move over to the birth chair again.

Uri sat behind her on a step stool. I sat in front of her on my milking stool. She started to push. Her waters broke; it was filled with meconium. Ugh. Not surprising for 43 weeks. I thought about asking Sarahle to come into the house but decided instead to raise the faith volume again. After all, Sarahle was just a shout away.

The contractions got stronger, and Tali's pushing became deeper. She asked me to come closer so she could push against me. Her hands were on my shoulders, then her forehead was on my forehead, and then her head was pushing against my chest, and then her hands were pushing on my head. When she pushed, I felt the effort inside my body. I heard the groans from her throat in my head. My head was bent forward, but somehow, out of the corner of my eye, I saw a dark area that looked like the baby's head peeking out. I reached down to feel with my hand, and glory be! It was the baby's head.

I asked Tali to move forward on the chair, and I slipped off of the stool and sat on the floor. One more push and the baby was born into my hands in a waterfall of meconium. She was screaming and crying, pink and gurgling. Tali took her up into her arms and immediately called her by her name, Noga, and comforted her. Uri was ecstatic. I was relieved. Tali transformed into a warm, cuddly personification of Mama-mush.

It was as if someone had hit a button on the remote control and changed Tali's channel. All the pain, discomfort, frustration and aggravation disappeared the moment that Noga came into Tali's arms. She was like a flash of warm, yellow light that lit up the room.

Lessons learned:
1. When a survivor of sexual violence tells me to go far away, it is a good idea to stick around. She might need me close by.
2. She who throws the sharpest arrows has the softest heart to protect.
3. Presence is a very flexible concept and has nothing to do with physical proximity.
4. Sometimes I need to be like water and flow with each woman and each birth process. Sometimes I need to be like the earth, soaking up pain, blood, guts and tears which women release as they move through their births. Sometimes I need to be like the sky, optimistic, light and full of options. Sometimes I need to be like a big tree planted nearby, sturdy and steady, waiting to be leaned on.

More Safety, Less Intimacy – Anat

Anat first came to me when she was in the 32nd week of her third pregnancy. Her first birth had been at home, but she described it as a disempowering experience. The midwife bossed her around in a manner that she remembered as hurtful. Her second birth was at a hospital with an epidural, an experience in which she reported feeling disconnected, both physically and emotionally. This pregnancy appeared to be normal except for the fact that in an ultrasound scan, the doctor reported having seen six fingers on one hand of the fetus. No functional problems were detected.

When I asked Anat about her past, she told me that she grew up in a violent household, and her father beat her from age four until about age eleven when she was big enough to run and not be caught. Her mother was passive and afraid of her husband. Her parents eventually got divorced. She felt that these experiences shaped her personality in many ways.

Anat has ambivalent feelings and reactions toward authority figures. On one hand, she is sometimes fearful, passive and submissive, and on the other hand, she can also be rebellious, angry and hateful. She uses dissociation regularly when she experiences fear, threat and danger. She is sensually hypersensitive and is very particular about audial, tactile and visual stimuli. She has serious difficulties with trust. She and her husband Yoav were members of a spiritual community for two years and were abandoned by its leader. This seriously aggravated her trust issues.

Anat was hoping for a different kind of birth experience this time around, an experience that would be empowering for her. She did not want to be managed by anyone other than herself and wanted to experience her birth in a positive light. I told her about my training in Somatic Experiencing, explained a bit of the theory behind it, and asked if she wanted to try a few sessions in preparation for her birth. She was happy about the opportunity, and we met four times.

During our second session, she revealed to me that in addition to having been beaten by her father, she had also been sexually abused by an uncle who, at first, had been a refuge from the violence of her father. We also talked about her perfectionism, her need for control, her need for approval and her fantasy of having the ability to become invisible, or at least to take up as little space as possible.

As the birth approached, Anat's level of anxiety rose. She was anxious about bringing another child into the world and about taking up too much space just by being pregnant and then by giving birth. She was afraid of the pain, and she was worried that it might trigger memories of other painful situations she has experienced, including her previous births. She was worried that she might not feel at ease at the birth center, knowing how particular she is about how things look, feel and sound.

She went past her due date and began to worry that something was wrong, as her two previous pregnancies had culminated on time. The days went by, and I felt her retreating from both me and the birth. There were fewer phone calls and several canceled visits. Finally, she came to the birth center for a check-up at 41+2 weeks instead of going to the hospital, the accepted practice. The monitor was normal, but her feet, legs and hands were very swollen. She had a few erratic contractions, but nothing that would indicate that she was nearing labor.

Anat was concerned about the fact that the birth wasn't happening, and was a bit anxious and upset. She was also confused and was trying hard to figure out what was wrong, whose fault it was and how she could make this birth happen. Her major concern continued to be that she was forcing those around her to make room for the birth and the new baby. It seemed to her as if everyone was busy with their lives and that she would disturb them by going into labor. During the last few days, her labor started and stopped several times.

We discussed options for encouraging the labor to begin. Other than acupuncture, she wasn't interested in using any other means. She went home to wait for labor to kick in, still frustrated and confused.

The next evening she called to say that she was having irregular contractions and that she and Yoav would like to come to the birth center. They involved the grandparents by inviting them to come to pick up the grandchildren. She was actively making some space for the birth. Yoav was hesitant to come to the birth center without evidence of strong, regular contractions but was willing to follow Anat's lead. He assured me when they arrived that her intuition is usually accurate.

They arrived at the birth center at around 10 pm. The contractions were irregular, every eight to ten minutes. She was three centimeters dilated, but the head was still high and the cervix was thick. She was certainly not in active labor. We all endorsed the notion that if she gave the necessary space and time to the labor, it would develop. But it didn't happen. The contractions got farther apart, and Anat got more and more anxious. She felt pressured to deliver the goods, to make this labor happen and it clearly wasn't happening. As time went on she became activated, and at one point she asked me to come into the bedroom and help her relax.

We did some SE-inspired work together, mostly grounding and re-sourcing, and slowly she was able to breathe more deeply and allow her body to relax a bit. It took a long time for her to get comfortable, but when she finally did, she just wanted to sleep. I was ambivalent about whether to stay the night at the birth center or to go home and sleep in my own bed. I didn't want her to feel abandoned, but I also didn't want to infringe upon her privacy and wanted to give her a feeling of security. In the end, I decided to sleep on the couch in the living room.

At around 5 am she woke up and came into the kitchen to get a glass of water. I woke up and stayed with her. Yoav was asleep. The color of the sky was just beginning to change from black to dark blue. We could both feel the morning coming. There were no contractions at all. We went outside on the deck and sat together in the dark.

Anat was anxious again; I could feel the tension in her body, her voice and her words. She felt she had screwed up by coming to the birth center without being clearly in the throes of active labor. She didn't know how to proceed. Should she go home? Should she try and induce contractions? Should she bring the children home from the grandparents? I suggested we let it be for now and decide in the morning. I made it clear to her that any decision she made would be acceptable to me. We both went back to sleep and woke up at 7:30.

Yoav went shopping and made breakfast, and afterward we held a team meeting to discuss the situation and the options. There were only two options: go home and wait for contractions to pick up on their own or try and encourage the labor to gain momentum with holistic methods. Yoav voted for going home and waiting for contractions. Anat wanted to stay and give birth. She had made the space for the birth and wanted to move forward. She understood that she needed a push to make it happen. We discussed different induction techniques, and she decided that she wanted to try homeopathy, together with massage and a bit of shiatsu.

I prepared two water bottles, one with Cimicifuga and the second with Caulophyllum, a standard, generic homeopathic induction. Yoav prepared a space for massage on a mattress on the floor with scented oil and relaxing music. We closed the shades and darkened the living room as much as possible. I read a book while Yoav massaged Anat's feet, legs and back. She took the homeopathy every 20 minutes. Within an hour she reported feeling contractions every four minutes. Her spirits were high, the contractions were regular and we all felt our moods improving.

Not long after that, I noticed Anat sitting outside on the deck crying. Yoav advised me to leave her alone. He said that she usually feels better after crying, and this would surely help her along in the birth process. The crying continued for about twenty minutes. She smiled at me, indicating to me that the crying felt good.

At about 10:30 Anat asked me to connect her to the fetal monitor on the deck. It was a surprising request, but I agreed. She told me later that she likes machines. During the monitoring she started to complain that the pain she was feeling did not feel like contractions, but was flu-like and located in her lower back and pelvis. She asked me to disconnect the monitor; she went inside to shower.

After a long, hot shower, she got into bed and complained of feeling chilled. She was under the covers in a fetal position and wanted to be left alone. I came in a few minutes later to take her temperature and found her asleep. I took advantage of the opportunity to go home, shower, change my clothes and reconnect briefly with the world outside of the birth center. The flu-like symptoms were confusing and irregular for birth; I took the time to think about it during my break.

When I returned about an hour later, Anat was up and about, still complaining about the aching pains and the chills. I took her temperature; it was 38.5, an actual fever. I was even more confused. Thoughts raced through my mind. What does this mean? An infection? A cold? Now? She had no other symptoms. Was the fever psychosomatic? I recalled her 20-minute cry and wondered whether she was experiencing an enormous emotional and physical discharge. I listened to the baby's heartbeat, and it was clearly tachycardic (very fast) between 170-180 beats per minute, a common fetal reaction to maternal fever.

I had many questions and very few answers, and I had to decide what the next step should be. After all, I am the captain of this ship, the conductor of this orchestra. I need to make the decisions when things veer out of the range of normal (I was a bit tachycardic myself). I called Maya. She made it very clear that in her opinion, we needed to transfer to the delivery room. Maternal fever is a reason for a transfer to the hospital with no room for opinions, analysis or deliberation. I was puzzled about the cause of the fever but decided that this was not the time to ponder it any further. I would think about it later.

I gave Anat an Advil to lower the fever and we discussed transfer to the hospital. I made a few phone calls to various delivery rooms which were all very busy. Poriya was the only hospital with some empty rooms. Within a minute, she was at the door, dressed and ready to go.

She didn't seem distressed by the idea of transferring and was anxious to get moving once the decision had been made.

We drove in separate cars. Anat and Yoav left the birth center first. I stayed a few more minutes to organize the place, close the windows and shutters, throw leftover food into the trash pail and organize a bag for the hospital. When I got into the car and backed out of the driveway of the birth center it suddenly dawned on me that it was Erev Rosh Hashanah, Eve of the Jewish New Year and that the road in the direction of Tiberias might be very crowded. Anat and Yoav were already on the way, and I wanted to suggest an alternative route with less traffic. Too late. They were already stuck in a bumper-to-bumper traffic jam on the main road.

I eventually reached the same traffic jam from a different direction, using dirt roads and shortcuts, but I was only about five kilometers ahead of them. Yoav also went off-road and followed my instructions to the shortcuts. The police stopped him for driving on the shoulder, and when he told the police officer that his wife was in labor, they received an escort to the hospital, sirens and all.

With all this, it took almost an hour and a half to get to the hospital. The car ride was Hell for all of us. I was terrified that the baby wasn't feeling well and was having difficulty dealing with his mother's fever. I could feel Anat's anxiety from miles away. I tried to call friends who could support me. Unfortunately, everyone was busy cooking and preparing for the holiday.

During my third phone conversation with Avner, about two thirds through the trip, I broke into tears. It felt like this was too much for me to handle. In their car, Anat and Yoav were also distressed. Anat stopped feeling fetal movements and was terrified that something had happened to the baby.

I arrived at the hospital ten minutes before they did, sat down on a bench outside the emergency room and waited, trying to calm down by telling myself over and over that everything is and will be okay. They arrived, and we went directly to the delivery room. When she told the midwife that she wasn't feeling fetal movements, she was hooked up immediately to the monitor. The baby was fine, still a bit tachycardic but showing clear signs of well-being.

As the strip of paper flowed out of the monitor, reassuringly documenting the baby's heartbeat, I could feel the tension melt out of my body. The baby is fine, and I could see that Anat was also relieved. Slowly her smile and sense of humor returned.

The midwives were kind and efficient. They admitted her to the delivery room by asking questions about the pregnancy, her general health and about what had happened during the last 24 hours. They were concerned about the fever, took blood and urine tests and gave her antibiotics intravenously. Anat was a bit overwhelmed by the bustle of action around her. She looked at me and said, "I can't believe I'm here. I ended up with everything I didn't want. I can't believe it."

There seemed to be some dissonance between what she was saying, her body language and her facial expressions, which expressed calm and well-being. I asked her to leave behind what she had planned and to examine how she feels, in the hospital, at this moment. She responded by telling me that she felt surprisingly good.

Dealing with the doctors was challenging. Anat was assertive in demanding time to make decisions at her own pace. I was assertive in stating my opinions, even when they were in contradiction to the opinions of the doctor. We fed off each other and paved the way toward creating an empowering hospital birth, even though it entailed Pitocin for induction of labor, continuous monitoring of the baby and antibiotics for the fever. Despite the physical restraints of the IV line and monitor cables, Anat was upright, active and moving. As the contractions started kicking in, she came to life, becoming more and more animated as the birth developed. She had no problem coping with the pain. She was rolling.

In the evening the fever returned and with it, Anat's disquiet and unwillingness to be tied down. She demanded to be released from the monitor and IV line and went into the shower. She stayed there much longer than the doctor had recommended but came out feeling so much better. She was having regular contractions and felt that she was finally in labor. She was going to give birth soon.

The doctor chose to ignore her contractions, insisted that she reconnect to the Pitocin and claimed that she wasn't progressing. At first, she protested and refused, and he demanded that she sign a refusal statement. She had no problem signing and somehow that made him even more determined to convince her to agree to renew the Pitocin. Then he sat down, took a few breaths, explained his reasoning in a patient, personal manner, and she agreed.

A half-hour after the Pitocin was renewed, the contractions got strong. Anat demanded again that the IV line and the monitor be removed. She wanted to go back into the shower. The midwife agreed, this time without consulting the doctor.

Five minutes later she was howling in the shower. I went in and found her naked and crouching in the corner. There was a puddle of water, soap, blood and secretions on the floor. She looked up at me and told me that the baby was coming. I felt her perineum and the head was pushing its way through her pelvic floor. I reinforced her feelings and told her that she is giving birth and that the baby is here. I called the midwife.

The midwife arrived in a bit of a panic. She wanted to move Anat into the bed. I told her that there was no time. I brought her a towel to provide a safe place for the baby to land. I turned the water off. Yoav arrived. Anat pushed once, and the baby tumbled into her hands. She was ecstatic. She looked up at us and said, "I did it. I did it. I caught my baby all by myself!"

We all took a few moments to recover from the excitement, and I led her back to the bed as she held the baby close to her chest. I assumed that the midwife would not be willing to deliver the placenta in the shower. She had had enough thrills for one shift.

The placenta came out five minutes later, and with it a larger than normal gush of fresh blood. Anat started hemorrhaging, and within moments the room filled with midwives and doctors giving her medications to help stop the bleeding. The bleeding was quickly arrested, and Anat was fine. I went home, and I was fine. The baby had 11 fingers and he was fine. Anat's fever disappeared, and they all went home the next day.

Lessons learned:
1. For a survivor of sexual abuse, a public space can feel safer than a private one. Intimacy can feel threatening.
2. The body can produce fever as a sign of distress.
3. Empowering births can happen anywhere. Home birth does not necessarily ensure a good experience.
4. I am thankful to be surrounded by a network of hospitals with delivery rooms, doctors, machines, medications and operating rooms. Home birth is only as safe as the medical support available when needed.
5. Challenges to coping with labor can have absolutely nothing to do with the level of pain of uterine contractions. Anat became motivated and energized when her regular contractions started to kick in. Not being in labor was more difficult for her to cope with than being in active labor.
6. The shower proves itself over and over again to be a surprisingly powerful tool that gently enhances the progress of labor.

Taking a Deep Breath – Ayelet

Ayelet is a survivor of abuse by her parents, primarily by her father. He was violent, verbally offensive and sexually provocative. Her mother was weak; she stood by and allowed bad things to happen. Ayelet sees her mother as a battered wife. Her brother claims that their mother sexually abused him.

Two of Ayelet's siblings left home before age 16. She tried to leave but stayed and became the first of her siblings to finish high school. She has little contact with her parents who are still together. Her father repeatedly amused himself by telling the repulsive story of how everything was filled with shit at her birth.

Ayelet's first birth was at Hadassah Hospital in Ein Kerem. She considered having a home birth but decided not to because she couldn't afford it. Instead, she planned a natural birth at the hospital with a doula, hopefully with no doctors, no instruments and no intrusions. At the time, she lived in the Tel Aviv area but drove to Jerusalem (60 km away) so that no one from her family would be in the vicinity, hovering or intruding on her privacy.

Ayelet and Or spent a full day together at home with the early contractions. They went to the hospital when the contractions became stronger and met the doula there. Ayelet's cervical dilation was small, and she was disappointed. She felt half-naked walking around in a hospital gown, felt negative energy from her doula and progressed very gradually from 1.5 cm. to 2 cm. to 2.5 cm. All she wanted was to be alone, but she was surrounded by all the people she didn't want to see, hear or feel: doctors, midwives and the doula. And, in direct contradiction to her request, her mother and brother also showed up. To this day, she hasn't forgiven them for being there when she fell apart.

The birth was long. She lost control, lost her desire to live and lost herself. She got to a point where she was suffering terribly, filled with anger and hate for the world. Eventually, she asked for an epidural at nine cm. She gave up. No one pressured her to take the epidural, so she could blame no one but herself. The opposite was true; they tried to persuade her not to.

After three hours of full dilation, Nir was born by vacuum delivery. It was a distressing reflection of her life, which she experienced as violent and disgusting. It sparked a profound, significant and troubling insight for Ayelet, that she had come into the world as a result of her father raping her mother. The labor room felt like a battlefield, littered with wounded and dead. It took months for her to recover.

Postpartum was a difficult time. She was sick, depressed, had problems with breastfeeding and suffered from yeast infections, hemorrhoids and parasites. After about three months, she began to feel moments of flow in her life. Nir developed into a significant resource for her. She is still surprised by how much love she generates. Through Nir, she is learning what it feels like to love and be loved.

Ayelet came to me during her second pregnancy on the recommendation of a doula, who knew I worked with abuse survivors. This time around, she wanted to give birth at home. It was part of her yearning for a healing experience. During this birth she hoped for movement, privacy, awareness, presence, love, breath, empowerment, cleanliness, simplicity, patience, femininity, serenity, joy and freedom. It was a long list, but its precision gave me hope. We met weekly, and slowly and methodically created a safe space for a potentially healing birth.

At first, I learned about her life, relationships, coping patterns, difficulties and challenges. Together, we discovered and explored a stubborn and toxic multi-faceted reaction pattern that lumped together disgust and hate, pushing people away, wanting to die and waiting for it to all be over. This pattern also dominated the unsuccessful manner in which she tried to manage relationships.

She explained how she is triggered into dissociation, and then we discovered together that she is often retriggered by the dissociation itself, creating a vortex that is difficult for her to exit. We came to understand how this problematic pattern prevents her from trusting people, forming intimate relationships, keeping a job and from finding her place in the world. Surviving is a daily struggle for her. For three months, we went through an enlightening therapy process together, taking apart the lump, one bit at a time.

We started by identifying resources at her disposal. Ayelet recognized a significant resource within herself, her ability to climb a steep, small mountain. As long as she knows that it doesn't go on forever, she can do it. This immediately brought to my mind the image of a fetal monitor strip, with one mountain after the next, one contraction after the next. This led us to fashion an approach to handling the contractions during labor, to climb one mountain at a time, one contraction at a time, knowing that birth does not go on forever.

We practiced the use of mindfulness and breathing techniques throughout the therapy process. Ayelet learned to stay with uncomfortable feelings and sensations, breathe through them and watch them change, instead of running away or disconnecting.

Ayelet shared with me her wish for a wise woman to enter her life. This woman would give her sound advice, hold and contain her, see her and hear her and be flexible enough to adapt to her changing needs. I wanted to be that woman for her. As the birth approached, Ayelet revealed more and more expectations. I became responsible for her not being retraumatized during the birth. I was in charge of keeping her grounded and feeling safe.

She wanted this birth to be clean, simple, empowering and healing. We worked hard to make this happen. Up until the last minute, we were both hopeful and afraid at the same time. We both understood that the birth could be an extraordinary opportunity for healing but also harbored the threat of disappointment and re-traumatization.

At the end of a session, we had an opportunity to test our relationship. Ayelet went into the toilet to urinate before going home. After she had already gotten comfortable, she realized that there was no toilet paper and she called out to me for help. I brought a roll, knocked, stood outside the door, waited and talked with her. I explained my plan, that I would open the door a crack, look the other way and toss the roll in her direction. She approved the plan, and I executed it. After she finished, she came out laughing and declared that this little incident had been absurdly significant. She suddenly felt deep inside that she maybe could trust me.

To make sure, she covered all the bases, and enlisted another support figure, Adi, a bodyworker and a wonderful woman. They met several times during the pregnancy and formed a close bond. The plan was for both of us to support Ayelet during labor.

It was Saturday morning. Ayelet called me at about 8:15 with contractions every three minutes. The contractions had started at about 6:45 and were gaining momentum. She wasn't sure that she wanted me to come, but I didn't heed her deliberations. I got ready and went, and I arrived at her apartment at about 10:00. I had already learned my lesson about how second births can be surprisingly quick.

Ayelet was on the bed and was having a hard time. The contractions were coming one after the next with very little rest in between. She seemed on the verge of panicking, and I focused on helping her change her state of mind. I talked her through the contractions, one at a time, and helped her to slow and calm down her breathing. I reminded her of the mountains, one breath at a time, one contraction at a time. It helped.

Adi arrived and continued calming her down while Or and I set up the birthing pool. He carried out Ayelet's orders, and tried to make everything perfect for her. Adi held her hand lovingly while they breathed together. She entered the water at 11:10 when she was six centimeters dilated. She thought I was lying when I shared this encouraging information with her, but I wasn't. It was beautiful, and it was true.

She felt better in the water. Her body calmed down, and the breaks in between the contractions became more significant. She was able to rest, catch her breath and drink some water. She used the breaks to tell us what to do to help her. Touch here, sit there, be quiet, talk to me.

At about 11:45 Ayelet felt some gentle pressure, and at noon she was fully dilated and started pushing. I ruptured her membranes because they were bothering her; she wanted to feel the head. The waters were clear. She pushed in several positions but couldn't settle on one that felt right. My feeling was that she would do better on land. I thought that gravity would give her a clearer direction.

A few contractions later, I suggested that she get out of the water, and she decided to move over to the bed. She started pushing on her side, but it didn't feel right either. She sat up, leaned back and allowed Or to hold her from behind, which in itself was a small miracle. At 13:03 she gave birth to a beautiful little baby girl. She couldn't believe it was true and couldn't stop saying it, over and over. Everyone was crying tears of joy and relief.

Her wishes for this birth had been: space, movement, privacy, concentration, presence, healing, love, cleanliness, simplicity, patience, femininity, empowerment, quiet, presence, breath, joy and freedom. It was all there. She had achieved the birth she had worked so hard for and deserved so much.

It all went by very quickly, and my only regret was that I couldn't record my thoughts during the birth. This birth was a victory for all of us. A good, simple, healthy home birth surrounded by loving caregivers was enough to make a big difference in one woman's life.

Since the birth, things have turned around for Ayelet in a big way. She can breathe more deeply now. She has learned that she has something to offer the world. Her heart has softened, her connections with her loved ones have changed and her mothering has been transformed.

Together, we have told the story of our connection to various audiences, including public health nurses, rape crisis center volunteers, midwives and therapists. Ayelet has become a doula and is now supporting other women through their birth journeys, using the lessons she learned to empower others.

Ayelet's birth raised many questions. How transformative can a good birth be? How can it positively affect a woman's life? Are these effects long-lasting or just fleeting moments?

It was my honor to participate in Ayelet's sacred process, and it is still my privilege to continue to ask these questions, having witnessed this birth and the ripples of healing it still generates.

Lesson learned:

1. The experience of accompanying Ayelet at her birth was very special for me. Every moment I learned something new: how important it is to remain in the present, how much breathing can help, how significant it is to be in a loving environment and how it is always possible that something new can happen.
2. I was thankful for the work we did together during the pregnancy. It enabled me to quickly identify Ayelet's moments of difficulty, answer her needs immediately and avoid unwanted experiences of dissociation. By talking to her throughout the birth, being super-present and providing unconditional love and support, I did my job and Ayelet never disconnected.
3. Ayelet filled me then and continues to fill me today, with inspiration. I learned from her that honesty, sincerity, courage and connection can overcome any obstacle that shows up along life's trail.

Riding the Horse – Efi

Efi came to meet with me during the 23rd week of her second pregnancy. She wanted to give birth at home this time because she didn't want to go anywhere near the hospital. Her first birth had been a negative experience. Her husband Noam was not on board with the idea of a home birth, and she didn't know how to bridge the gap between them.

Efi was 32 years old when we met. She described herself as physical; she does sports, rides horses and knows her body well. She was a student of the Elboim Method, a body-based therapy modality. She works with children with cerebral palsy through therapeutic horseback riding.

Efi tends to ask questions about how she manages herself and her family: the food they eat, the type of education she favors, and the way she manages their health. She does not take the middle path; she has a nonconformist streak. Her partner Noam is exactly the opposite. He is the source of stability and support in their life together, and he tends to trust large organizations like the government and the health care system. He believes that the safest place to give birth is in the hospital.

Efi described her first birth as complicated. She had prepared to hire a doula but decided not to in the end. She and Noam did a birth preparation class together and then moved to a new house two days before she went into labor. She went to the delivery room with a birth plan in hand which basically said, "Leave me alone!"

The birth started with the spontaneous rupture of her membranes and contractions. Her labor was intense and painful, but her progress was slow. After hours of contractions with minimal progress, the midwife in the delivery room laughed at her birth plan, ridiculed her, and told her that she would never be able to survive a natural birth.

She took a very long shower; Noam was with her. The contractions seemed more manageable, and when she returned to her room, her cervix was four centimeters dilated. She was exhausted and asked for an epidural. Within two hours she was fully dilated. She understood that her stress had been slowing down her progress.

Her second stage was long and arduous. She was told over and over that she wasn't pushing properly and that there was fetal distress. She was also told that she had to get the baby out or have a vacuum extraction. After nearly an hour of intense, directed pushing and an episiotomy, baby Adi was born blue and flaccid with her umbilical cord wrapped three times around her neck. A pediatrician was called in.
Efi asked him questions about the baby's condition and received no real answers. Adi was taken away to receive respiratory support. Efi cried and cried. All she could think of was the children with cerebral palsy with whom she worked.

Noam did not help and support Efi as she had expected. She partially blamed herself for this, as she had pushed him away every time he tried to approach her. Her mother, who was also with them at birth, became overwhelmed and retreated within herself. Efi sent her home after the epidural. She gave birth feeling defeated, angry, scared, alone and disappointed, mostly in herself but also in all those who are closest to her.

When we started unraveling the events of her birth, some major issues presented themselves. One issue was her need for control. She used her relationship with her horse Black to describe how she felt. There is an element of fear in horseback riding which she loves to conquer. She knows Black's power and capabilities, his size, weight and speed. But the reins are in her hands, and the reins enable her to control his power. Together they become a team; they work together; they communicate. Under her body, she feels his strength; on his body, she feels her own power. Within a year from the day that he became hers and they became a team, they became national champions. Together they are a powerful and successful duo.

During the birth, she lost the reins; she felt out of control and overwhelmed. Her horse had run away. In addition, she felt mocked and ridiculed by the midwife's derisive and sarcastic comments. In retrospect, she understood that all of this had triggered a memory of sexual abuse during her childhood and a feeling of abandonment.

During the birth, when none of the people she was relying on were emotionally available to defend her against this abuse, she felt rejected and alone.

Other issues that emerged were her love of competition, her ability to fight and her need to win. She planned the birth as a runner prepares for a marathon. She searched for ways to conquer the pain. She thought that if she closed herself off to the pain, she would be able to survive it and win. The contest was between herself and her body, and she was determined to succeed.

As the labor progressed, her birthing body became the enemy. She felt under attack, and she tried to push the contractions away. The derogatory words of the midwife stimulated her to need to compete, to do better, to win the battle against the pain and the midwife. Deciding to ask for an epidural was her moment of defeat, of failure. She was disappointed in herself; she had lost the competition; she was a loser.

She knows and appreciates that in order to succeed, she needs the support of a loyal and wise coach, someone who knows her and loves her. When training with Black, Efi's riding instructor communicates with her through her glance, her tone and her words, especially when the going gets tough. During the birth, she received no such coaching, neither from Noam, her mother nor the midwife. She had no one to turn to for help or advice. After the epidural, communication with the midwife was easier; full dilation followed soon after.

When it came time to push, Efi was sure she could do this well. Her body was strong and capable. All she needed was someone to guide her, to tell her exactly what to do. Instead, she was reprimanded for not pushing well and doesn't remember receiving any explanations that could have helped her do better. She heard her body being cut, She was told that the head was out, and suddenly Adi was on her belly, blue, floppy, not crying. The midwife was worried and nervously asked Noam to call out for a pediatrician. Noam did as he was told and yelled out. Efi was frozen with fear.

The pediatrician arrived and cared for Adi, while Efi asked him repeatedly if the baby was going to be OK, trying to gain some information. He yelled at her for asking too many questions. After she explained that she works with kids with CP, he answered abruptly, "We can't know anything right now." Then he was out the door with her baby in his hands.

Then the doctor who had told her that she didn't know how to push sutured her. She felt defeated in all aspects of this battle. She felt abused. Her power had been depleted. When she got up to go to the bathroom several hours later, she fainted.

The scope of our exploration began to widen beyond her birth. Efi was beginning to gain some new insights. One day she brought up the topic of fear and explained to me that she knows two kinds of fear. The first kind includes the fears that everyone experiences like going on a giant roller-coaster, bungee jumping or riding on a fast horse. These are the fears that she knows how to overcome. All she needs is something to hold on to.

And then there are the fears that seem irrational and illegitimate, the things that scare her the most, like darkness, sleeping alone in bed, sudden noises, sudden touch and sometimes sexual intimacy. When she said it out loud, she realized that she was again pointing to the possibility that she had been sexually abused. She shuddered to think that this was the case but understood that it could explain the fears that felt so irrational to her.

That same day, she told me that she had decided to give birth at my birth center. She knew that Noam would not agree, and she had not discussed it with him yet, but her mind was set; it was going to be.

The next time we met, she wanted to explore the connection between pain and fear. Between meetings, she had come to an understanding that the pain of her contractions had triggered an irrational fear, a fear that couldn't be conquered. It was too much for her to handle. When we tried to pinpoint the moment in the birth when she felt that it was too much, she remembered the words spoken to her by the midwife just before she went into the shower. A moment before she decided on the epidural, she said to her, "Your behavior is unacceptable. You must calm down, and now."

These words triggered a thought and then a memory. She understood that she was stuck, and that there was no way out of this situation. No one was going to help her. She found herself in a room with no door, a place with no exit. It was no longer the delivery room. It was her grandfather's storage shed. With tears rolling down her cheeks, she turned to me and asked what her grandfather's storage shed was doing in the delivery room. It made no sense, and at the same time, it made way too much sense.

One week later when we met again, Efi was filled with additional information about her grandfather. She needed to know more; her memory had opened up. She remembered that she hated going to visit him. She remembered that his house was filled with pornographic materials. It became evident that she had some history that needed exploring, but she was less than ten weeks from her due date. Together we decided that this was not the right time. We decided to concentrate all our efforts on preparing for the coming birth, and if issues arose that were related to the abuse, we would deal with them as they surfaced.

Efi connected with an online community called Active Birthing. She read inspiring stories and watched videos that brought her to tears. She went to a meeting and listened to stories told by women who gave birth at home. It sounded logical to her. She drove home and told Noam that she wanted to give birth at home. At first, it didn't go well. One evening, they watched the movie *Orgasmic Birth* together. Early the next morning, he left her a note saying: "Everything will be OK. I love you. We are in this together."

The next time we met, Efi announced that they had decided to give birth at home. Noam would be coming to meet with me, and together we would discuss what that meant for all of us. In her mind, she was beginning to formulate a birth plan. She was thinking "yes" to water, soft lighting, intimacy with Noam, trust, letting go, breath, being touched with permission and being helped. She was saying "no" to closed spaces, silencing herself, fear of abandonment and pleasing others. She wanted to go through the birth on her own power and give birth feeling just like she feels when she is on Black's strong back.

The meeting with Noam went well. He asked questions about equipment, emergencies and transfers. He needed to hear the answers in order to feel safe and fully supportive of Efi. Home birth would not have been his choice, but he was committed to supporting his wife more successfully this time. He knew that he had let her down the first time, and he wasn't about to let that happen again. Our next meeting was an intake. I was excited. I felt that this was a very significant decision for Efi, Noam and their relationship.

At our meeting the following week, we had a long talk about her fears. We then used her fears as a reference point, imagined the opposite and created positive affirmations. She took these sentences home and fine-tuned them until they were perfect. She then printed them and placed them in strategic locations all over the house. She immersed herself in positive thoughts that challenged her fears.

At our last meeting before the birth, Efi chose three goddess cards as sources of inspiration for the birth. For her head, she chose Pachamama, the goddess who gives women the confidence they need to give birth. She knows about life, birth, death and growth. She told her, "You can give birth." For her right hand, she chose Artemis, who steadily holds her bow and points her arrow. She sets her goals in a very clear manner and then lets the arrow fly to hit its mark. For her left hand, she chose Eurynome, an ecstatic goddess with huge white wings representing freedom and capability. She went home with the knowledge of a basic, powerful and simple truth, that women know how to give birth.

One day after Efi's due date, her waters broke at 2 am, at first in the form of a slow drip. She tried to rest. At 5:00, there was a gush of water, this time with light contractions every 10-15 minutes. The next phone call was at 6:45; the contractions were getting stronger and closer together. By 8:00 Efi was experiencing strong contractions every four minutes. She sent Noam with Adi to the kindergarten and asked me to come to join her. In the meantime, she did the dishes in the sink, straightened up the house and washed the floor.

I arrived at 9:00 and found Efi on the birth ball coping with strong contractions every three minutes by breathing through them. The living room was decorated with her affirmations; there was a photograph of Black on the wall near the pool. I examined her an hour later, and her cervix was four centimeters dilated. She was talking and telling jokes so we all knew that she was in a good place. My instructions from her were to boost her spirits only if I saw her showing signs of weakness. This was clearly not the case. Efi noted that at this stage in Adi's birth, she was already defeated and with an epidural.

Efi wanted the pool to be available to her, so we filled it up. She decided to enter it and luxuriate in its warm waters, glancing over at Black every once in a while. Within an hour, her cervix was six centimeters dilated, and within another hour, eight cm. I telephoned Dikla at noon; she was to be our second midwife, and it was time for her to come. The next hour was difficult, but Efi battled through it, allowing herself to receive support from all three of us. At 1 pm she was fully dilated and pushing.

I couldn't hear the baby's heartbeat in the water, and I couldn't tell if it was the baby or the Doppler, so I asked Efi to step out of the pool. I anticipated that this was going to be a difficult transition for her, but was confident that she could handle it. I needed to be sure that the baby was OK. Dikla whispered in her ear that she could do this.

Efi bent her knees and went into a deep squat. Dikla and Noam supported her while I prepared to catch the baby. I could see the head, and I told her so. She didn't believe me, but then at 1:19, the head slipped out together with a chubby little hand. The rest of the body followed. Nitay made his entry into the world, and Efi was ecstatic.

Noam was moved to tears. He was filled with admiration, appreciation and awe of his powerful wife, the woman who takes him places he would never dream to go by himself. Efi was overjoyed that he had been brave enough to trust her and allow his heart to follow hers. It was a very special moment. Efi was so glad that she had given her body a second chance and allowed it to prove its knowledge and capability.

Three weeks after the birth, Efi brought Nitay to meet Black. They became friends immediately, both honorary members of Efi's fan club.

A few years after the birth I invited Efi to tell the stories of her births to a class of midwifery students. I was lecturing on the topic of home birth, and I asked her to present her perspective. She was able to summarize the lessons she had learned about the differences between home and hospital birth. This meeting allowed her to contribute to the education of these new midwives. Straight from her heart, she asked them to be kind, listen and support their clients and not to ridicule, abuse or yell at them.

A year and a half after the birth Efi returned to my clinic seeking assistance in uncovering more pieces of the puzzle of her past. Her journey through the discovery of her abuse history was underway. She also felt, for the first time, that she wanted to spend a lot more time in the company of women. She took a course to become a postpartum doula. The experience was both empowering and healing.

Efi then participated in a support group sponsored by the Rape Crisis Center, wondering all the time if she was in the right place, among these women, in this circle. Participating in the group convinced her that she did belong there. She then took a course to become an on-call volunteer for the hotline.

Efi created a unique business that combines her two passions, horses and women. She wanted to pass on to other women the sense of empowerment she had achieved through her experience with Black.

Lately, her friends have begun asking her to accompany them to their births. Today she is a doula.

Lessons Learned:

1. I learned from Efi what it means to be courageous. She has the uncommon ability to know what she needs, to act on her instincts and listen to her intuitions. Even though the finish line is often uncertain, she continues to walk her path. She feels what she needs to heal herself and in doing so, enables those walking beside her to also heal.
2. The discovery of a repressed sexual assault shakes the ground on which a woman is standing. It takes time, courage, patience and a lot of support to touch these painful materials. The search for the truth leads to the release of irrational fears. In place of the fear, there is a renewed sense of freedom.
3. Over and over, I am thrilled to discover how one significant life resource, like Black in this story, can have such a strong and positive effect on other, seemingly unrelated areas of one's life.

Orly The Lioness

Orly first came to meet with me during the 35th week of her second pregnancy. She wanted to give birth at my birth center. She had considered a home birth during her first pregnancy but decided, in the end, to have the baby at Poriyah Hospital in Tiberias. Her partner Sa'ar trusted her to know what was best for her and was supportive of her decision to give birth outside the hospital this time.

Orly teaches dance and yoga at a studio that she owns. Sa'ar works with youth, preparing them for army service. At the time we met they were living in an apartment in Orly's parents' house on the family farm. She made it clear to me that having the baby at their present home was not an option.

Orly's first birth was neither long nor difficult. Seven hours after her waters broke and her contractions started, she gave birth naturally at the hospital. This made her a terrific candidate for a home birth. Her first and foremost request for the approaching birth was to be in control. She asked not to be touched without permission and to catch the baby herself. I asked her if she had ever been attacked or abused. "Yes," was her clear and straightforward answer. Between the ages of 12-16, she had been sexually abused by one of the workers on her father's farm.

Orly had kept the story from her parents for many years, and when she was in the 6th month of her first pregnancy, she decided it was time to reveal the truth. Orly and Sa'ar felt that this secret was affecting their relationship and that it was time to open the issue in the hope it would allow them to move forward with their lives. They assumed the worker would be fired when her parents learned what he had done and that he would be out of their lives forever. It was especially important to them for him to be gone before the baby arrived.

There was an initial conversation with her parents, and then the discourse continued via numerous heated discussions and written correspondences. Her father's response was unsympathetic, and the worker wasn't fired. Her parents didn't believe her story; they told her to find a way to come to terms with whatever happened and to get on with her life. She was shocked.

Orly and Sa'ar continued to live on the farm, exposing Orly and her daughter Noga to this man. She continued to feel threatened by him and continued to experience the parental neglect from which she suffered as a teenager. I understood why she didn't want to have this baby at her home. It was not a safe place.

Orly's pregnancy was more or less eventless. We met three times, having initiated the connection at 35 weeks. Orly was sweet and open. She knows her body well and seemed very confident about her ability to give birth. Sa'ar was very supportive and loving. His admiration for his wife was apparent in both his verbal and nonverbal communication.

The birth started during Orly's 39th week. At 7 pm she called to report that she was having contractions every ten minutes. The next call was at midnight, and it was from Sa'ar. The contractions were coming every four minutes, and they were on their way to the birth center. She arrived with a cervical dilation of five centimeters and was experiencing regular, strong contractions every four minutes.

We filled the tub, and she went right in. The warm water was soothing and relaxing; she stayed in the tub for an hour and then moved over to the bedroom. By 3:45, the contractions were stronger, more intense, and coming every three minutes. Her dilation was seven centimeters, and she returned to the tub. An hour and a half later, she left the tub again with a cervical dilation of nine centimeters and went back to the bedroom, supported physically and emotionally by Sa'ar every moment of the labor.

By 7 am she was fully dilated and pushing. At 7:35 her waters broke, and at 7:44 Nitay came into the world and into the arms of his beautiful mother. The second stage was difficult for Orly, but she did it, and she earned her victory. This birth was about the same length as her first, maybe even a little bit longer, but most important of all, it was over, and her sweet baby was here, safe in her arms.

Two years later, Orly lost a baby at 24 weeks; she was devastated. A week later, with broken hearts, they left their home and Orly's birthplace. It was saturated with her painful history of abuse and neglect. They moved to nearby farming community into a small house of their own that was free of ghosts. They wanted some peace and quiet and to live somewhere where no one knew them. Less than a year later, she became pregnant again. Nitay was now three years old; Noga was six.

Early in our first session, it became evident that it was important for Orly to begin processing the events surrounding the stillbirth.
One main issue was her loss of confidence in her body. She had been feeling fine and did not sense that anything was wrong with the baby.

One day, her mother mentioned that her belly seemed small, and when she asked her if she had been feeling the baby move, Orly realized that she hadn't been paying attention during the last few days. With the kids in the car on their way to a picnic, they decided to make a stop at the hospital to ensure that everything was OK.

From that point in time, everything that happened was a blur. It all happened so quickly, too quickly to grasp. The fetus was without a pulse, and Orly was immediately admitted and induced with Pitocin. Sa'ar took the children home. This left Orly alone in the hospital. Within 12 hours her womb was empty, and she was weeping.
She didn't hold her dead baby, a decision she regrets deeply. It was all over, yet she didn't feel ready for it to end. She hadn't had ample time to process anything of what had just happened.

The stillbirth left her feeling out of control and disappointed in herself and her body. The second stage was particularly troubling for her, and parts of her memory were missing. She suspects that she disassociated. She remembers having no idea of what to do, how to behave or how to help herself during this ordeal. She was lost.

Both Orly and Sa'ar took time to heal after the stillbirth, and they deliberately didn't rush into another pregnancy.

In looking retrospectively at all three of her births, she concluded that she has very different emotional reactions to the different stages of labor. She understood that she is good at coping with the first stage. She knows how to deal with pain and suffering, something she learned through years of absorbing neglect, disappointment and abuse. She can breathe through whatever pain is sent her way, coping with it in whatever manner seems fitting at the moment. It is a passive experience; she knows how to suffer passively, to find a way through difficulty until it passes.

The second stage is a different ball game. It demands that she be active, assertive and upright, stating her needs and working hard to get the baby out. This is not her forte. She tends to lose her power and freeze. Her anger feels like that of a 12-year-old, paled by frustration and powerlessness. The second stage confuses her, and she gets lost when it shows up. She doesn't know what to do; she loses connection with the primal survival instincts of aggression and action, instincts that where stolen from her by her abuser.

For the upcoming birth, Orly's wish was to regain her confidence in herself and to give birth at home. Because of her fear of the second stage, she felt that she needed a plan. She knew that she could overcome her fears if she could acquire some confidence and some tools. In most areas of her daily life, she is highly capable. She runs a dance studio; she is a gifted teacher, choreographer, dancer and organizer. When she tapped into these capabilities she could see them as resources, and we used them as a basis for the beginning of the reconstruction of her confidence in herself as a birther.

During our next meeting, I invited Orly to tell the story of the stillbirth again, this time with the help of therapeutic cards. I find that telling a difficult story through a right-brain channel helps to create a sense of order in the jumbled memory of the event. New understandings tend to surface and crystallize. At first, her choice of a vast myriad of cards reflected that she was feeling overwhelmed and confused by a mumble-jumble of emotions and memories. After arranging and rearranging, adding and subtracting cards, she was able to create a visual storyboard of the stillbirth with a clear and distinct beginning, middle and end. The speed of the events continued to feel problematic, so Orly opened up some space between the cards on the table. This created some time and space in between the events. I suggested she try and imagine what she would have done differently if she had more time, more space, and more breath.

She envisioned that in between learning of her baby's death and the onset of the induction, she would have gone outside with her children for a few hours, sat on the grass with them and explained to them what had happened. She wouldn't have allowed Sa'ar leave her in order to take the children home. Instead, she would have asked someone to come to pick them up. In between the breaking of her waters and the delivery of the dead fetus, someone would have told her what was about to happen, and she could have prepared herself. Instead of allowing the midwife to take the baby away, she would have taken him into her arms, held him, looked at his face and felt the weight of his body. She allowed the gaps to fill themselves in. She took a doll into her arms and felt the satisfaction and relief of completing the movement that her arms had yearned for ever since the stillbirth. As she held onto the doll, her body relaxed and her breath deepened.

When she looked back at the cards on the table, she wanted to take the negative cards away, and so she did. The only one she left on the table was a card representing the fear of death. She created a circle with supportive cards around it, but it wasn't enough. She went back to the deck and searched for a new card that would be powerful enough to challenge the fear of death. She found her card; it was a lioness perched on a bluff. This lioness knows how to protect both herself and her cubs. She knows what courage is. This lioness touched Orly in a very deep way, and as time went on, she continued to help Orly to connect with her courageous self.

The next time we met, new and old fears showed up again. The second stage continued to confuse and scare her. She was unable to look at pictures or movies of women giving birth. When she tried, she felt her entire body cringe in sheer terror. Orly decided to bring in the lioness for support, for she sensed that the lioness knows how to give birth as do all female animals in nature. This helped, but she needed more. She needed some practical tools and physiological explanations, which I was happy to provide. The combination was a good one, nutrition for the mind, the body and the spirit.

At our next meeting she was still ambivalent about birthing outside the hospital. Birthing at the birth center would provide her with more freedom, flow and movement, but it also required that she face her fears and recruit her courage. Birthing at the hospital would be more clear-cut and simpler. There would be no emotional processes that would need to take place. We parted that day without a decision regarding the intended place of birth. We both knew that when the labor began, she would know exactly what was best for her. The lioness within would help her decide.

I received a call from Orly on her due date at 6:30 am. Her contractions had started two hours earlier and were now regular, every eight minutes. The plan was to get the kids up, dressed and ready and to take them to nursery school. They arrived at the birth center at 8:40 with contractions every five to seven minutes. They went for a walk, rested and had lunch. I went upstairs to my home to give them some space. We all agreed that she needed some time to get into the right frame of mind.

By 2 pm the contractions were getting stronger and closer together; they were coming every five minutes. Two and a half hours later the contractions were every four minutes, and her cervix was six cm dilated. Orly was on the birth ball, in the shower, on hands and knees, standing, swaying, breathing and connecting with her inner strength. She placed the lioness card on the kitchen counter, in sight and available for inspiration and confidence.

As the contractions became stronger and pushing felt imminent, she moved with the lioness into the bedroom. She went down to the floor, leaned forward on the bed with her upper body and asked Sa'ar to prop up the lioness card on a pillow in front of her, in clear view. In between contractions she stole glances at the lioness to remind herself what she is capable of.

At 7 pm her waters broke, she was fully dilated and pushing. Ten minutes later, her beautiful baby girl cub Gefen was in her arms. She was so proud of herself. She had chosen to go through the process and face her challenges. We bore witness to Orly overcoming her fears, right there, before our eyes.

There was a true knot in the umbilical cord which was also coiled around the baby's neck. She survived the birth courageously just like her lioness mother.

A year later, Orly, Sa'ar and their three children moved back to her village of origin, but this time into a home that did not belong to her parents. She felt strong enough to go back and reconnect with her neighbors and friends without becoming overly involved with her family. She and Sa'ar set very clear boundaries; these enabled Orly to feel safe and protected. In the meantime, the worker had been fired.

Two years later she became pregnant again. When she came to see me she was in her 31st week, and the nation and the world were deep in the throes of the COVID-19 pandemic. Both she and Sa'ar lost their sources of income, and they were at home with their three young children around the clock. Her anxiety level was rising, and she could feel it eating away at her confidence. At the time, I had already retired from doing home births, and this was contributing to her anxious state. She felt deflated. She said, "I don't have the strength to deal with this. I'll just go to the hospital."

When we explored this statement, it reminded her of a behavior pattern from her childhood in which she would throw away the cards in the middle of a game. She didn't want to play if she couldn't win.

She didn't feel that she had the energy or motivation to get to know a new midwife, open up to her, expose her vulnerabilities and deal with the complexities that Covid-19 brought to the table.

She went on to share with me that she now understood that she had dissociated during the second stages of all of her births, including the last one and that she is still afraid. When I asked her what the lioness had to say about all this, she realized that the lioness had been asleep for several months. As we continued to talk and discuss her options, she felt the lioness wake up, raise her glance, stretch her back and begin to explore the surroundings.

One week later when she came back for a second meeting, she looked different. She reported feeling as if she had woken up from a deep sleep. She wanted to discuss her options with Sa'ar again, this time not from an attitude of throwing in the cards but from a place of informed consent and free choice.

She opened up all her options: in or out of the hospital, at my birth center or at home with a new midwife, with or without a doula, at this or that hospital. She remembered the feeling of knowing that whatever she decided would be the right decision for her. She could feel her confidence filling the empty spaces within, but she still wanted to understand her stubborn fear of the second stage and her history of disconnection. It was still an obstacle to her desire to trust herself.

We did a micro investigation of the sequence of events and made some discoveries. When the sensation of fullness in her lower pelvis starts, the fear emerges, sparking a reflex to contract her pelvic floor to protect herself. At the same time, she knows that she needs to open up to let the baby out. A conflict of two diametrically opposed actions arises, opening and closing. This causes her to want to run away, disassociate and escape the conflict. She knows that she needs to remain present in order to give birth. This causes another polarization, another inner conflict. She can't do what needs to be done, pushing, because she is so filled with inner conflict. Her body wants to contract and escape. Her mind tells her that she needs to open up and remain.

She understood that the key to creating a new way of being and a different reaction to the second stage was by facing her fears head-on. Orly made a long list of all of her fears. Together we imagined their opposites and turned each one into a precise and positive affirmation. She continued this work at home, and she created an expansive and very specific list of exactly what she wanted to be thinking and feeling during the birth. She plastered the walls of her house with these lists and practiced saying them to herself several times a day.

- I will give birth in a place where I feel safe and comfortable.
- I will give birth at my own pace.
- I will ask for and receive everything that I need.
- Sa'ar and I will take care of ourselves and we will be taken care of.
- I allow myself to escape and come back and forgive myself if I do so.
- I accept the feeling of the pressure of my baby's head.
- During the contractions, I remain present.
- I allow myself to open up.
- I trust my body.
- Everything is for the best.
- I know precisely what to do.

Orly planned to bring the list with her to the birth and have Sa'ar read the affirmations to her whenever she needed a boost of self-confidence. They decided to birth at the newly renovated L&D unit at HaEmek Hospital in Afula. She stayed home as long as she could, and Sa'ar read the affirmations to her as per her request. An hour after they arrived at the hospital, she gave birth to baby Tuval. Finally, she felt that she had conquered the second stage, and this meant so much to her. This time she was an active participant, and the lioness within vigorously pushed her baby out into the world and into her waiting arms.

Lesson learned:
1. Orly's path of healing has a dynamic, ever-changing life of its own. Sometimes she runs along a clear, open track in leaps and bounds; sometimes her pace is slower and heavier, barely moving forward. Sometimes it is like a roller coaster, going up, down and all around, with loops, dips and some very scary curves. Sometimes it feels dangerous, and the path is cloaked in a thick fog. Sometimes, it is a difficult, uphill climb with a clear and obvious trail. The key to her process has consistently been to remain open to the possibility that healing is possible, face the challenges as they present themselves and never give up.
2. Our insistence on exploring the minutest details of Orly's experience paid off and enabled the magic of healing to occur.
3. The lack of my physical presence did not weaken Orly at her last birth. The opposite was true; she had a chance to explore the impact of the process we had gone through together. My heart was joyful from afar.

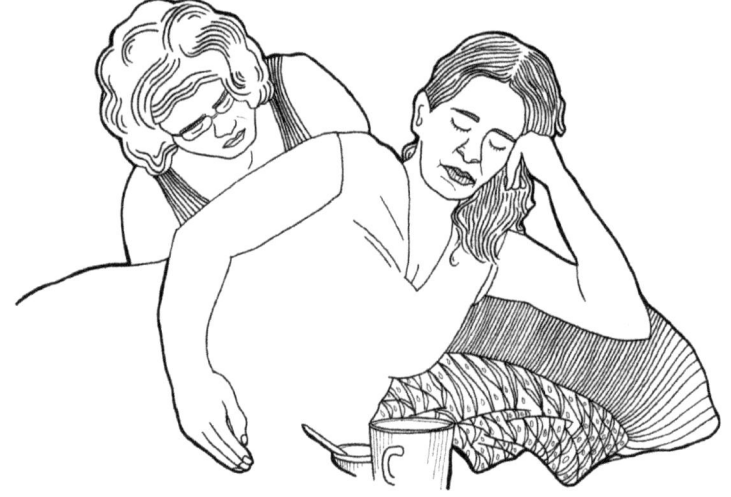

Winding Down – The End of an Era

After 15 years, continuing to attend home births developed into a question mark. Being on-call 24/7 started to become challenging and sometimes even annoying. My body was screaming out, begging me to stop torturing it with sleepless nights, a broken biological clock and the constant stress of endless uncertainty. I had to reevaluate my priorities. I had to choose between home birth and me. This time, for the first time, I chose myself.

I set a date. I declared that I would not take on any new women whose due dates were beyond June 1. My kids and grandkids were coming to visit from abroad, and if I stuck with my plan, I would be free to be with them and enjoy their company all summer long without looking at my phone and hoping it wouldn't ring. I was excited about not being torn between two things that I love, my children and my work.

No one believed that I would go through with it. I had threatened to stop several times but hadn't been able to carry through with the plan. I hadn't been ready enough. This time felt different. I was more at peace with myself; it was time.

I had no grandiose plan the next step would be; no one had offered me a great job. I firmly believe in making space for the next thing by allowing the emptiness just to be and not rushing in to fill the void. I finally had an opportunity to practice what I preach.

I didn't experience the emptiness until the summer ended, but I felt it very powerfully when it hit. Something was missing. The requests for home births continued, and I had many opportunities to get used to the new words that were coming out of my mouth, "I don't do home births anymore. I have retired." It sounded like someone else's voice speaking someone else's words.

I felt myself transitioning to the next phase of my life. The question that occupied my thoughts more than anything else was how to go forward without the home births and still answer my deep and basic need to be significant. I had a long talk with my wise daughter Yael about this. When she heard the crack in my voice that always comes right before the tears, she stopped me and said, "Ima, you have been so significant in the lives of so many women. The time has come for you to take a well-deserved rest."

This was all I needed. Finally, I was ready to take on the next challenge, even though I didn't yet know what it was. I was ready for a challenge that didn't require getting up in the middle of the night, committing to sleepless nights and striving to cope with the ultimate uncertainty that is called birth. Maybe I didn't need a new challenge. Maybe I could just sit back, relax, rest and reflect. At least for now.

One Last Story – Gal's #3, My #444

Late in January, I received a text message from Gal, "Where are you in May? Save me a spot. My due date is May 16." This would be two weeks before June 1 – just in time. In a flash, I understood that Gal's birth would be my last before retiring. We set a date to meet, opened a file and began her pregnancy follow-up.

Gal saw on my face that I had something to tell her. She is super-intuitive and nothing goes by her unnoticed. I told her of my plans to retire and that her birth would be my last. Her reaction was a mixture of disbelief, relief and worry. The first two were expected and apparent – doubt that I was actually retiring and relief that she managed to slip in before the ax fell. But what was the story behind the worry? She worried that because it would be my last birth, there might be some drama around that, and it would be more about me than her.

She was right to be concerned about this, and I took her message to heart. I promised her that I would do everything in my power not to let it become my story. It was her birth, not mine. And I asked her to keep an eye on me and say something if she saw me losing my direction.

We have known each other for over six years. This was to be Gal's third out-of-hospital birth with me; the first two were at my birth center. She and her husband Shaked recently moved into their brand-new house in their kibbutz, and this time around, she wanted to give birth in her own home.

When I first met Gal and Shaked, I was very impressed by how much space Shaked created for Gal, how much he respected her and how he thought the world of her. In our discussions, if I asked him a question, he repeatedly referred me to Gal, saying, "Gal knows; ask her." I wasn't sure if he was avoiding participating in the conversations or if he really did feel that Gal was a source of great knowledge, wisdom and intuition.

When I witnessed Gal birthing, it all came together. She was one of the most emotionally intelligent and attuned birthers I had ever encountered. Her first and second births were smooth and eventless, her second much quicker than the first. She gave birth exactly on her due date. She used the knowledge she had acquired from Hypnobirthing and spent most of her births breathing quietly, gently moving and relaxing. She was truly inspiring to be with; she made birthing seem so natural and unassuming. After both births, we joked that if she could market what she has, she could probably make a lot of money.

This pregnancy was also healthy and normal. At first, the placenta was a bit low, but that worked itself out. Gal was tired and almost anemic but she fixed that with an iron supplement. Her glucose challenge test was a bit high, but the 100gr was normal. Everything was fine and good. We had agreed on "no drama," and we were each going to do our part. Gal planned to give birth in her bathtub.

The contractions started on the morning of May 15, the day before her due date. I was at a meeting with some home birth midwives from Imahi, and they heard my phone conversation with Gal. They knew that this would be my last birth; I practiced minimizing the drama with them in preparation for my meeting with Gal and Shaked.

Late in the afternoon, she lost her mucus plug. At 6 pm she called to report that she was having irregular contractions ten minutes apart. At 9:00 she and Shaked went for a walk, her contractions got stronger and they asked me to come. I was aware of the fact that I was going to my last birth, but I didn't allow myself to bring attention to the story.

On the way, I made several phone calls in an attempt to find a midwife available to join us. No one was free. For a moment a thought went through my mind that this could turn out to be a problem, an issue, the drama that I dreaded – that I would be alone at my last birth and something horrible would happen. I got a grip on myself, took a deep breath and decided I would solve this when I got to their house, and not while I was driving.

I arrived at about 10:00 and found Gal with regular contractions every four minutes. She asked me to examine her – her cervix was dilated five centimeters, 90% effaced and the head was still high. The contractions did not warrant her focused attention, and she declared that she was going to sleep and suggested I do the same. I even got my own bedroom. Before I dozed off, I managed to find a midwife from Nahariya (Roni) who was willing to come and join us but on the condition that I would let her go home in time for her morning shift at the hospital. Good enough. Roni had all four of her babies at home and was a firm believer.

A little before 3:00, Gal woke up with stronger contractions every three minutes. Her cervix was eight centimeters dilated, and the head was coming down. We filled the bathtub with warm water and she got in. I called Roni. After she arrived, the contractions got even stronger, Gal's waters broke, and at 5:13, Gal and Shaked welcomed their third beautiful daughter into the world. Her umbilical cord was wrapped around her legs twice, and she took a minute or two to pink up, but she was just fine.

I had my eyes on the baby and the mama, and Roni had her eyes on me. She knew that this was my last home birth. I felt her scanning me, looking for signs of emotions. I was fine. I wasn't thinking about myself. I had promised Gal that she would remain in the center of my focus, and I held up my end of the deal.

Later, after Roni left and Gal and Shaked got settled in bed, I decided to get back into bed myself and get some sleep instead of driving home. The last thought I remember before I drifted off was how thankful I was that in 15 years, in 444 births, I had never lost a baby or a mother. Thank God and the Goddess.

Lessons learned:
1. I was glad my last birth was with Gal. She knew how to stand up for herself and demand that I keep her in the center of the story. There would be plenty of other opportunities to celebrate the end of my home birth career.
2. Gal's birth also gave me a chance to experience, for the last time, the power, simplicity and wisdom of a woman giving birth in her home, in her territory, on her turf.

Later that morning, after breakfast with Gal and Shaked, I drove home with a new sense of lightness. As I pulled into my driveway, my friend Leslie called to tell me some horrible news. Her son Asaf, who was living in Las Vegas, was hospitalized and needed emergency surgery. She had to drop everything, hop on a plane and go to be with him. She had planned to attend an international conference in Vancouver but had to cancel everything. She wondered if I knew someone who could take her place at the conference.

I thought for a minute or two and answered in the calmest and most collected manner that I could muster up at the time, "I'm free." A week later I was in Vancouver, starting the next phase of my life. There I met amazing people from all over the world, doing all different kinds of significant work to improve the lives of women. I was inspired. Maybe I'll go back to Africa? Maybe I'll create a non-profit? Maybe I'll write a book? Everything seemed possible.

Epilogue – Dear Duggi

Deganit, also known as Duggi, was my muse while I wrote this book. She helped me realize that I could successfully put my thoughts into words if I just put my butt on the chair and my fingers on the keyboard.

The number 444 keeps showing up in my life. I often wake up in the middle of the night, and when I glance at the clock, I see that the time is 4:44. I have been told that it is a good sign, "an angel number" and that my angel is using this number to show me that she is with me, reminding me to feel confident and supported.

Duggi, my angel, has inspired me in many ways. I was with her when she gave birth at home to three of her five lovely children. We shared a platter of sushi in the hospital, five days before she died. We had many opportunities to talk, get to know one another, disagree and agree. We were a part of each other's lives for eight years.

Duggi had enormous amounts of knowledge in numerous fields. She had strong opinions and something to say about just about everything. She was smart, talented, creative, funny, dedicated, hard-working, determined and above all, loving. She knew what was best for herself and her family and went about achieving it. Watching her doing so was inspiring.

Deganit and her husband Howard made Aliyah in 2010 with their son Jojo when Deganit was pregnant with their second son Yaron. When they first arrived, they lived in Carmiel, a development town in Galilee. A few years later, they moved nearby to Eshchar, a residential community in Gush Segev and made it their home.

They lived in various rented apartments in Eshchar until they finally built their own house. Each birth took place in a different venue.

Duggi's first two births were in hospitals, one in London and one in Israel. It didn't suit her. She did not like to be poked and prodded. She had her doubts about the feasibility of conventional medicine, and she loved researching her options. I am honored that Duggi chose me to be her midwife three times. It was a stamp of approval, virtually a certificate of excellence. She was very particular.

I started writing about Duggi's births because, after all, this book is dedicated to her, and then I stopped, hesitated and gave Howard a call. I asked him whether or not, to his knowledge, she had written anything about her births. He referred me to her voluminous and hysterically funny blog entitled, *"Diary of an Aliyah-nik."* Instead of doing my best to recall and recreate Duggi's births, I decided to let her speak in her own voice and quite a voice it is!

The first two excerpts were written in 2010 after Yaron's birth, her second hospital birth and her first birth in Israel. Here the foundation was established for her decision to give birth at home.

The spellings are British, for example labour, not labor. When I read her words, I can still hear her voice with that beautiful accent.

It's a Boy! (Obviously) 7 September 2010

So, after our lovely night out with friends, I felt confident that they would be able to look after Jojo when I went into labour, so the following morning (Friday) that's just what I did.

Woke up just before 7, got everything ready, awakened Sleeping Beauty [husband], and called a cab. We got to Ziv hospital at around 8:30 and by about 9am I was holding my beautiful teeny baby son. Clearly, the Lord thought what with our rather stressful Aliyah, it was the least He could do. Thanks for that.

All was fine, although I would NOT recommend going through the transition stage in the back of a taxi going up the bumpy windy road to Tzfat hospital. For anyone who doesn't know, "transition" is that dreadful part of labour when the woman suffers the most, in other words, the bit where she starts shaking and yelling obscenities at anyone unfortunate enough to be around her (in the movies, it's usually the opportunity for the funniest line). I thought I was rather calm actually, I only asked the driver about 15 times how long until we got there, and I only asked him to overtake twice. (Bit of a problem as I don't know the Hebrew word for overtake). Of course, my luck, we were stuck behind the only slow driver in Israel on a one-lane road.

It was a beautiful view though, which was very calming. Only it was a bit difficult to stay calm as when I arrived the doctors/nurses/midwives/ bloke on security (not really sure who was there, as not really paying attention) were running around like headless chickens. I don't think they had ever seen a woman in the final throes of labour before. Which is a bit surprising. At one point I even heard some bloke saying "Mah Karah?" in a sort of "Now what seems to be the problem" type manner. Erm, let me think. Woman with a large belly leaning against the reception counter groaning. Let's have a think....

Anyway, they were all yelling at each other, wondering what to do with me. The chap at the front had attempted to wheel me in a chair (wasn't having that – why would anyone imagine that to be comfortable??!) and I ended up walking the corridor until they threw me on a bed and wheeled me up to the maternity unit, yelling at each other loudly in Ivrit (Hebrew in Hebrew), and ignoring my requests for my husband. (He had to sign in. Even in a crisis, Israel maintains high levels of bureaucracy. Priorities....) Nobody bothered speaking to me in a calm, controlled voice or asking me any questions (at least I don't remember them doing that).

It seems I had upset their protocol and now they were a little unsure as to what to do. In the end, I just let them get on with it. I discovered long ago that the best way to deal with shouting Israeli people is to just ignore them.

The midwives were ok, barely had time to examine me between contractions as I was basically ready to go, and my doula didn't make it until after the birth (when I first called her at 7:30am, I told her not to come yet, as it didn't seem so bad). Not one of them spoke a word of English, but in some ways that made it easier to focus, and I could do exactly what I wanted. I would recommend that to anyone with a baby on the way, birth seems to go a lot smoother when you are allowed to listen to your body.

Anyhow, sprog 2 is small, weighing 5 lb 11 at birth, but healthy and very sweet. Looks just like the first one did so I keep calling him Jojo. He is a very considerate baby, allowing everyone a good night's sleep before his arrival and causing no trouble at all. Eats when he is supposed to, burps when he is supposed to, contented. We knew it was a boy all along, despite never finding out. I have always had this feeling we will be one of those noisy all-boy families that nobody wants to come and visit because the house smells of feet.

How to Survive an Israeli Hospital – 8 September 2010

- *Number of cockroach sightings: 0 (Come on, it's not that bad! Israel is a developed country you know!)*
- *Number of schnitzels consumed: 5*
- *Number of nurses spotted who have walked straight out of the 1950s: about 17*

Tzfat hospital. Beautiful mountain views. My window looked onto the stunning Kinneret. Brand new, almost-finished maternity unit. Lovely birthing rooms (not that I got to hang out much in there, shame coz there was a jacuzzi....) Kosher meals 3 times a day. Bliss.

Well, yes, all that stuff is great but the problem is the general philosophy of the place is still dreadfully old-fashioned and the nurses must be hideously underpaid as they seem to suffer the same issues as Israeli waitresses, i.e. they are doing you a favour if they bring you something. Over the course of 3 days, I attempted to ask for pain relief for my frozen shoulder, hot water and perhaps an herbal tea bag for my dreadful cough that was probably driving my poor roommate mad as well as myself, (why do hospitals think that new mothers want to drink caffeinated drinks??!) and various other straightforward things. They were all met with a "are you mad?" look, and I realized pretty quickly that this was a DIY hospital. If you ever want to get out, you have to do what you are told and look after yourself. Heaven knows how the C-section women cope. And goodness knows I saw a lot of C-sections. For a modern hospital, with natural birthing facilities, I was shocked at the number of women I saw recovering from them. Perhaps it just feels that there are more of them as they stay in for longer, but still, the high number did not reflect well on the skill of the midwives.

I noticed this immediately after the birth when they offered me drugs to "shrink my womb and quell the bleeding" (er, doesn't that just happen anyway??) I asked about it and they said: "Oh well you know after a long labour, it's often very necessary." I blinked at the midwife in surprise –

has she not been paying attention? I had only been in there for about 45 minutes! (In fact, the friends we were staying with were in total shock when we called them, saying that they hadn't even managed to complete one laundry cycle in the time it took me to give birth…) I explained to them that after a natural birth, I didn't feel the need to spoil things with unnecessary drugs. They also gave all sorts of things to the baby (after promising he would only be gone for a few minutes) some of which were probably not necessary, but I hadn't had a chance to research this so I let them get on with this. They are supposed to be at the forefront of medical science here, after all.

There was, however, one lovely midwife named Hila who actually apologized to me afterward for trying to change my birthing position, saying she wanted to help. I thought that was very sweet, and there was a nice English – speaking nurse who apologized for the confusion regarding: taking the baby away and helped me translate what the others were telling me to do. This was especially handy as one of the nurses GAVE MY CHILD FORMULA WITHOUT MY PERMISSION!!! I kid you not. After they harassed me, I agreed to give him one tiny boost as he was small and yellow, and I knew he would be fine without it, but the nurse told me I would never get out of there if I didn't…. then I asked a nurse to take him to the nursery during the night for his jaundice test, as I was feeling a bit dizzy giving her strict instructions NOT to give him a bottle. But when I got there, it was too late, they had given him a big dose. I screamed at the nurse and ran down the corridor with the cot in tears. I couldn't believe the betrayal of trust there. Of course, the formula knocked him out for hours so I couldn't feed him, which was very uncomfortable. I gave them hell for that and the doctor told me he had reprimanded her. I should bloody think so.

I could not believe the number of newborns on formula and sucking dummies. Nor the hilarious policy that the babies had to be wheeled around in cots (they are worried you might faint when you carry them about, which is kind of understandable but not so relaxing to hear these trolleys trailing up and down the corridors day and night).

They also wake you up in the middle of the night if your baby is found (Shock! Horror!) in your bed (can't they just quietly put it in the cot and let you sleep, like in Watford General?) and to take your temperature and blood pressure. They don't see the need for new nursing mothers to get some sleep. At one point I woke up in the middle and gasped loudly in horror at the ghostly apparition that appeared before me. Turned out to be an Arab midwife telling me to put the baby back in his cot. Somebody had the bright idea of giving her a matching head covering for her white uniform and, being the middle of the night, I assumed that she was the ghost of a previous nurse.

Most upsettingly, the nurses didn't seem to understand anything about the basic mechanics of breastfeeding or bonding with one's baby. The funniest was a nurse who came to check on me on Shabbat afternoon. I had been nursing the baby who passed out on me, so I left him snuggled on my lap whilst I read my book. The conversation went something like this:

- *"Why are you holding your baby?"*
- *I wasn't sure how to answer this one. So, I gave her what I hope was an incredulous look and said: "Because he is my new baby."*
- *"Shouldn't he be in his cot?"*
- *"Er, no, he is very cozy on me."*
- *"But his neck looks awkward."*
- *"I think he was probably more squished up in the womb."*

Sigh. I can't believe in 2010 a nurse would still believe that a baby is better off in a cot than on his mother!!!

I hoped Shabbat there would be relaxing, what with it being a religious hospital, but all that meant that there were billions of people around, as it was the weekend. I shared a balcony with the next room and on Shabbat afternoon I had 2 Arab men sitting outside my window with a full view of my hospital bed. That wasn't fun. On Sunday I had to tell someone to stop smoking!! For goodness' sake. They were pretty militant about visiting hours, so I guess they used the balcony as a hiding place. On my final day there (I discharged myself in the end as I felt I could do more for the baby at home than they could with their monitoring) a lady was wheeled into my room following what I presume was a C-section. Her Russian husband and parents were quietly taking care of her when all of a sudden, a tall man in a uniform and tattoos stormed in:

- *"Mishtarah!" (police) "You need to leave now!" (directed at tiny Russian new grandma sitting by her daughter's bedside)*
- *Oh my gosh! I think. This must be a drug raid! Perhaps she is storing drugs in her daughter's labour bag! Wow!*
- *"But I am her mother" the woman pleads. "I am taking care of her"*
- *"NO! YOU MUST LEAVE!"*

They were kicking her out as it was 2 pm, and there are no guests between 2 and 4. I could not believe the way they treated the poor woman. They also tried to hustle us out even though we were packing up, and the nurses were pushing past us trying to make up the bed, even though we tried to explain that it would be easier if they let me, my husband, my son's buggy, the car seat and the new baby's cot exit the room first. But they didn't get it. Most of them were really miserable and moody, and the only cheerful staff I saw there were the cleaning ladies, who probably enjoyed this part of their rounds the most, as it was a brand-new wing with lots of cute new babies.

Anyway, here are a few tips for anyone planning to give birth in Ziv hospital:

- *Bring your own herbal tea bags.*
- *Get a window bed. Or grab one as soon as it's free.*
- *Press the red button if you want something, don't go to the nurses' station. They are more confident in droves.*
- *Avoid avoid avoid Russian nurses. Racist but necessary.*
- *Ignore the doctors. Ok, maybe that's a bit harsh but take what they say, imagine you live in a mud hut in Africa, and ask yourself, "Is it really necessary?"*

- *Be very direct about your requirements. If your Hebrew isn't 100% ask an Israeli to tell them or search for the one English-speaking midwife/nurse/doctor.*
- *Have a birthing plan and stick to it (within reason). Shout if necessary. Or do as I did, and pretend you don't understand them when they tell you to lie on your back.*
- *Say no to drugs. Seriously, I have never seen people so willing to hand out drugs. It's worse than Kings Cross.*
- *If you have an Arab roommate, asked to be moved. Again, this is not a racist thing but their families do come to visit in packs and you will feel like you are in a scene from My Big Fat Greek Wedding when all you want is to relax with your new baby.*
- *Learn to love schnitzel.*

The next three blog posts were written by Duggi after her third, fourth and fifth births, all three of which were home births. Each birth took place at a different house; only the fifth in the beautiful house that she and Howard built in Eshchar.

Call the Midwife – On Home Births in the North of Israel
3 March 2013

Despite me praying that this baby would not roll up before I recovered from whooping cough (yes, I was lucky enough to get that in my last month of pregnancy, and wasn't it fun coughing away), we had finished moving house (lucky me again). Once again, I have not made it to 38 weeks. My babies routinely reach around 2 and a half kilos and my body decides it's time to go! I had read countless articles about babies "knowing when the mother is emotionally or physically ready" but still, he couldn't wait. So much for that plan!

Towards the end of week 37, I had mild contractions whilst preparing for Shabbat and on and off over Shabbat, but nothing painful, so I carried on. The contractions didn't start to get noticeable until after Shabbat, and as my midwife predicted, they didn't hot up until the kids were in bed. I have heard of home-birthers who set up viewing stands for their kids to watch the birth process, but this seemed deeply wrong to me. I don't think it's something small children need to see – who wants to watch mummy suffering??!

After Jojo had stayed up watching nature programmes with us (both kids sensed something was up, and we had read "There's Going to Be a Baby" in preparation with them most of Shabbat) Husband spoke again with the midwife who decided to ignore my "it's not happening yet – ow – no they're not so regular" and come anyway. Good job she did. She came around 9pm when I was happily watching Dancing on the Edge on my sofa. I still thought it was a bit early to call her, but she examined me and announced I was around 7cm dilated. I seem to do birth quite quickly. Anyway, I was happy on the couch for another hour or so whilst Husband and Midwife bonded and prepared the upstairs room and birth pool. The Midwife asked for my permission for a trainee to join her, which I was happy to do. I went into the pool around 11pm, and was happily in my Zen mode with candles and a lovely CD from a friend of mine, except for the hideous coughing between contractions (very painful, but may have made the baby come faster). It was a far more pleasant experience than my hospital births – no one barking instructions at me, everyone trying to support me (rather than panicking about silly things like beeping machines), all in all quite tranquil. I find music very powerful in its ability to transform my mood. In the same way, I find the noises of a hospital very stressful, and after my last 2 birth experiences, I have a deep distrust of medical interventions in labour. Let me clarify – I am not anti-doctors or anti-hospitals; I just think there is a time and a place for medicalization). Of course, the last hour was a bit hairy – this was labour after all – but I felt safe with Husband and Midwife close by and I don't think you can feel this level of safety with strangers.

My son Raviv turned up soon after 1am. I found the birth pool a relaxing place to be, the water seemed to take the edge off the contractions. I was pretty tired from the birth and the coughing, but being at home felt more "natural" to me – for want of a better word. He was placed in my arms straight away – my smallest baby yet – and everything was calm, unhurried, no dragging him off for checks or prodding and poking. Nobody forced me to take drugs in order to deliver the placenta (which Husband buried the next day, fun for all the family). I called my parents soon after, as it was getting late in the UK and I knew they had to catch a flight the next day, so I called to tell them the news – when they asked me what the baby weighed, I couldn't even tell them, we hadn't got to that part yet. All very calm. (He was 2.4 kilos in case you were wondering). All I could tell them was that he was a boy.

Then I got to relax on our sofa bed whilst the midwife and Husband busied themselves clearing up, examining the placenta, filling out a few forms… and after a couple of hours, I took a shower and had the pleasure of climbing into my own bed. Bliss.

The next morning, my 2 "big" boys were up bright and early and came running into our room. Then they saw the baby in his basket and they stopped dead in their tracks, eyes popping out of their heads. "The baby!"

They were so happy. And on the bed were 2 wrapped presents for them – stuffed dolphins (from the baby of course) since they had both thought the sonograms "looks like a dolphin". It was a lovely morning. I think it was nice that mummy was home, nobody had to schlepp to hospitals or feel that mummy was "unwell" or they were somehow out of the picture.

Husband tried to take Jojo to Gan but he didn't want to stay there, he wanted to come home and join the action, and I can't say I blame him. A new baby is a huge family event, and I think the early weeks are very important in how the siblings accept and respond to the baby. So far so good. They are slowly learning what Gentle means! And they love him very much.

Our midwife came to check on us a few days later, and the children's doctor from our clinic kindly visited us for no charge – a service he performs presumably as his way of supporting home births. I am surprised the government does not promote them; they would surely save a lot of money. But that's for another blog. Amazingly, my little baby put on weight in his first week.

Frequently Asked Questions

So many people responded to my home birth by saying "Oh I would love to do that but I am too scared" or "that's my dream" or acted as if I was some sort of hero, (strange really, as I truly find hospitals far more frightening) so I decided to write this list of FAQs for those considering a home birth. It's really not that big a deal.

Isn't it a bit messy?
Not really. In hospitals, they leave all the clean-up until the end, so it looks like a crime scene. In reality, it's not so messy at all (mine certainly wasn't) and the midwives deal with it all as it happens. No big deal.

But isn't it dangerous?
Here's the tricky one. The reason a lot of women opt for a hospital birth even though they would prefer the environment of the home. Assuming both mother and baby have been checked out – no obvious problems, no anemia, nothing wrong with the fetus that may require hi-tech medical care, then the chances of something going wrong and the midwife not foreseeing it are very slim. To quote one of the many books on home births and the like which I read during pregnancy, most birth emergencies can be seen looming ahead by an experienced midwife.

And of course, the chances of the mother/baby needing medical care in the first place are drastically reduced by having a home birth (if you don't believe me on this point, check the statistics. You will be very surprised).

Don't you need to (legally) see a doctor?
A pediatrician should see the baby within 36 hours. It does not have to be in a hospital. We had a lovely local doctor pay us a free home visit.

What if you decide you want pain relief?
As far as I know, midwives don't bring any pain relief with them. I used a TENS machine right at the beginning, for a few contractions, but to be honest, this only helps with back labor. I found the water more helpful (you can't have both for obvious reasons). So, if pain relief is important to you, I wouldn't recommend a home birth.

What if you have a big baby?
I did extensive research into this and I couldn't find any link between long/problematic labours and big babies. I have 2 friends who have home birthed some huge babies, with no reported issues. My midwife actually commented that smaller babies can cause more issues as they can get stuck (mine did, the last 20 minutes were pretty tough). Women are designed to birth the babies they have (and it's not a competition)!

How do you find a midwife/doctor?
I went on recommendation from good friends.

What if there is an emergency?
Ambulance. I packed an emergency labour bag just in case. A decent midwife will pack you off at the first sign of trouble (this rarely happens). Most of the terrible news stories you hear of births that went wrong involve a mother/baby that was high risk or an incompetent midwife. Or more likely a couple that was not planning a home birth!

How much does it cost?
Not a cheap option. Especially if you factor in the lack of money from the hospital (this goes down with each child you have, so we didn't bother collecting ours). Luckily, I have a father who hates hospitals as much as I do so he was willing to help.

Do you need a doula?
It is handy to have the extra pair of hands, but it's another expense. I have a wonderfully supportive husband who could fulfill the handholding role, but If I didn't have him (or an alternative) I would hire one.

What if you live in a tiny house/flat?
We lived in a tiny house, it's not a problem. If you want a water birth you need to make sure there is space for a birth pool, and somewhere to put the kids! We had a room upstairs which we used and they didn't wake up.

What if the baby needs help?
My midwife turned up armed with oxygen. From what I know most serious conditions are now detectable in the scans. So, it's unlikely you would be caught out.

What about the mother's recovery?
This is the only potential downside in my opinion. If you are at home, you see the housework that needs doing. So, unless you hire some cleaning help, it can be quite hard to ignore. I found myself doing laundry on Day 1. (Don't try this at home). Luckily, I had friends who kept coming over and telling me to rest. But if you are a house-proud person, beware.

It's a Boy! (again) Home Birth No.2 11 March 2016

After what seemed to me like a very long pregnancy – the first time I actually made it to 38 weeks – I went into labour on a quiet Friday night. I have no idea how anyone makes it to the full 40 weeks. I was starting to get severely p*ssed off. Having reached a date exactly between my No. 1 and No. 3 child, I felt this would be a good time. I sent Husband off to bed because things were moving slowly and not terribly painful. My contractions warmed up through the night but seeing as it was Friday night, I felt strange turning on the TV. So, I just went to bed. My midwife offered to come, but for some reason, I wasn't convinced I was in labour.

Around 5am, I started to experience real pain so I told the midwife to come. When I called her, my phone read 4 degrees as the outside temperature. The thought flashed through my head: "I cannot imagine going to a hospital right now. Getting up from my cozy bed, putting on clothes, walking down our stairs into the cold, Sitting in CAR (ugh) and bumping along to a hospital 45 minutes away, full of bright lights and noisy staff..." What utter hell. I have no idea how I had my first two kids in a hospital, or indeed how anyone does it.

My midwife rolled up around 6am but by this point, I was too far along for the water birth I had planned. It takes time to blow up the pool and fill it. I have no idea why I left things so last minute, but when she examined me I was already 9 cms. dilated so that was that. No floating around in the water for me. But at least I got to stay in bed on a Shabbat morning... a rare treat! Soon after my kids woke up and I was now at the most miserable point – transition I suppose – and wondering how they would cope with the news that mummy was having a baby, but it was fine.

Mornings are a cheerful time for them and they were excited by the idea. Jojo got his younger brothers dressed, put coats on them, grabbed a jar of granola, marched them up the road to our friends' house, and announced that mummy was having a baby. Luckily the friend had been warned. So, all was good. (Jojo later informed me that he had peeked into my room and saw me on the bed in pain, and he felt sorry for me. How sweet.)

After that my labour progressed pretty quickly, I always feel better when I know my kids are in safe hands. And number 4 was born at 8:30. No trauma for my kids of mummy rushing off to the hospital. They just got to play in the park for a couple of hours or so and when they returned, they found sweet little Yakir in a basket surrounded by 3 little wrapped gifts – toy trucks and a tank. They were thrilled. (Although I suspect Yaroni was hoping for a sister…. Luckily, he got over it when he saw how sweet the baby was). It was all strangely mellow. We explained the gifts were from the new baby and they were very happy. My midwife and her assistant (they always work in pairs) hung around to sort out the paperwork and check all was well. Lucky for me it was Shabbat… so I had food for the entire day all pre-prepared, and we got to have a nice kiddush with our midwives.

We had planned to bury the placenta and plant a tree nearby but as we haven't quite moved into our house yet, my lovely midwife had the bright idea of freezing it. Unfortunately, she didn't label it so hopefully, I won't accidentally defrost it for a stew one Friday night….. "Placenta anyone…?"

I assumed my children would not really think that the gifts had come from the baby, but it seems I was wrong. Later that day as I sat on my balcony holding my new baby and watching the kids playing outside, I heard a long and earnest conversation between Yaroni and Jojo discussing exactly how the baby got their presents ready. How he got up at 2am and found the cello-tape…. so I now understand how children believe in Father Christmas. It's definitely more fun believing in a little magic now and again.

I, of course, had my own little magic. Having a baby on Shabbat is a slightly magical experience. (A little sad though, as you can't take photographs. Still, the memory is forever immortalized in my head). So far, all my babies were born on weekends, but only this one turned up on Shabbat itself. Aside from that, I am sure my landlord was happy. Instead of having my kids riding their toys around our house from the early hours of the morning, they were all out the door by 7am. So, they would have had a quiet one, their first in the 3 years since we moved in…

A Girl? You Can't Be Serious 12 May 2018

My reaction to the arrival of our first female baby was more or less the title of this blog. I asked the midwife to turn her round to make sure it wasn't a boy. Dead serious. Unlike 99% of Israelis (who are not known for their patience), I decided to keep it a surprise. I was pretty sure it would be another boy anyway. The pregnancy was the same, except I think she kicked harder than the others.

The labour went pretty well, all things considered. I usually have babies on weekends (yes true) but I had to wait for a friend to have hers, as we were sharing a midwife. I went to my belly dancing class one evening around 37 weeks and the girls told me they were sure I would drop the next day. Well, I did wake up with mild contractions plus I had that strange urge to do lots of housework.

I sent the kids off to school and told Husband to stay home in case I went into labour whilst caring for Yakir (age 20 months). I decided I had better cook lunch and dinner because I didn't fancy starving after giving birth and having Husband offer scrambled eggs. So, I made a tortilla for lunch, almond burgers and brown rice and homemade sweet and sour sauce for dinner, and a fantastic loaf of sourdough seed bread, which I have not yet managed to recreate. It's funny how I will forever associate that food with having a baby.

This time we gave our midwife more notice (mostly because we love her company) and called her shortly after the kids got in from school. She rolled in around 4 pm, drank a strong cup of coffee and promptly fell asleep on our sofa. As only a midwife can do.

The older boys went off to their after-school activities, Raviv went to play with his girlfriend over the road and I decided to do some belly dancing. Great distraction. Eventually, things got more uncomfortable, so I migrated upstairs with the midwife. The boys came home and were sent to the neighbour's for dinner. Around 6:15 or so I got into the bath and the baby arrived by 7. I had made Husband promise he would hold my hand throughout and not check his phone.... except he had to text our neighbour to instruct how much Insulin to give Raviv during my final contractions. But we can forgive him for that one.

The bath is an amazing place to have a baby if you like taking baths. Plus, it's a very easy cleanup. I highly recommend it.

We sent for the kids as soon as I was settled back in bed, so they got to watch the placenta examination, the baby being weighed and checked. Each had a cuddle. They were only gone about 2 hours in total, which was terrific for them. No scary being whisked off to various places while mummy disappears.

Happily, my midwife had the other new mum to visit in our village the next morning. Another friend on my street had a baby girl the same morning, so the girls on my street group were already Whatsapping when I decided to announce mine. (They were all in shock that I had given birth without anyone noticing...was I expected to scream deadly wail) Anyway, in the end, my midwife stayed overnight, which was very fun for us as my kids consider her one of their adopted grandmothers.

The boys were very excited to have a sister, although I think Yakir was in shock. For about 3 months after the birth, he woke up seeming surprised and thrilled that she was still there. He has named her RahRah after the noise she makes when she cries and the name has stuck. She has since become the center of all the love in this house and a sort of doll for everyone to play with. Yakir is incredibly gentle with her and is a trusted babysitter as much as the other boys, despite being barely 2 years old.

Since this was our first opportunity to celebrate the birth of a baby without the trauma of an operation (brit mila-circumcision) we decided to throw her a big bash. I had three rules, no impersonal speeches, no boring beards, and no bows on the baby. My friend Nirit filled our entire downstairs in decorative pink laundry, I hired 3 separate ladies from my yeshuv to do the food, and people brought stuff too. We named our baby girl (officially) Sienna Rivka and invited friends to give blessings. The boys prepared a fantastic show. This included Jojo serenading the baby, Raviv serenading me, and the Fairy Tale Story of her arrival in

English with Hebrew translation by Yaron. The fairy tale ended with a rousing jazz dance performance by my oldest 3 boys. After doing 4 brits, 2 of which we had to hold in shul on Shabbat/Yomtov, it was great to finally throw a party in our own special style. I sang a song of thanks accompanied by our friend Eran on the piano, who then led the audience in his own version. It was all good fun.

Two years later, Deganit got sick with a bad virus that swept through her house. She got sicker and sicker and eventually was hospitalized with severe pneumonia which led to organ failure and her tragic demise. She never went home to her beautiful children.

My Eulogy at Deganit's Funeral

On Wednesday morning, after Duggi was readmitted to the hospital, I was on the train when she wrote to me and asked me to come save her, that she felt very weak and anxious; and that she felt like she was dying. I tried to calm her down, and explained to her that I was on my way to Tel Aviv, and that today she was going to have to save herself
(as she has always successfully done in the past, with Howard by her side). I made some suggestions regarding soothing music, positive thinking and grounding exercises, and she wrote back that she was listening to Rachmaninoff. That sounded a bit dramatic to me, and not very relaxing, but she insisted on Rachmaninoff.

Today I understand that she understood what was happening. She knew that she was dying and that she knew what she needed (as always). She needed strong, emotional music that spoke straight to her heart, because she was a woman who lived through her heart – a heart filled with so much emotion: so much love, so much sorrow, so much hope (and now) so much fear. She needed to hear strong music that could echo all of this.

And her heart was also filled with so many plans: books to write, music to play, songs to sing, dances to dance, delicious foods to prepare, cakes to bake, parties to plan, projects to create, trips to take. She certainly wasn't planning on leaving us. Of that, I am sure. She had too much to do. I am sure that she is as shocked as we are to be gathered here today, maybe even more. Because this was not the plan, she always had a well-worked-out plan.

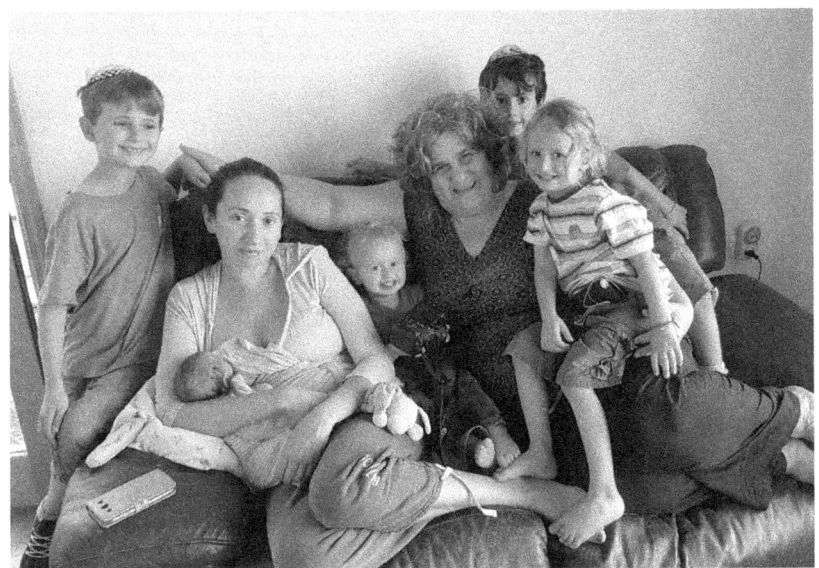

Where does this leave us? This leaves us with many precious memories of a very special woman, a woman who was both smart and sensitive, creative and resourceful, courageous and cautious, perceptive and intuitive, and devoted to her family in ways that only those who knew her and witnessed her dedication could understand.

And what will happen to us? We will miss her terribly and mourn our loss. There will be many days when we will feel that this tragedy is irreparable. And eventually, we will adjust our lives, and we will vigorously try to fill in the gaping hole that she has left within us. And we will fill that hole in with love because only love can help heal this wound.

And that is what she would want because she lived her life precisely in that way – where the solution to every challenge was to love her beautiful family as vigorously as is humanly possible and do what was best for them. And we will make it through the days, one at a time, loving each other, loving her memory, and seeking her wise advice by asking ourselves "What would Duggi do?" And she will live on through us via the wisdom she imparts upon us. And every day we will be thankful to be alive and to have each other, and we will miss her.

Acknowledgments

This book received the loving support and encouragement of an entire village – my village: my family, my friends, my teachers, my sister midwives, and my clients, along with all the talented and dedicated women who helped me along the way. If I were to attempt to name every one of you personally, I would probably forget too many, so I choose to let each of you find yourselves within the categories mentioned.

I am grateful to everyone who read the text and got excited, made suggestions and fueled my motivation to continue to write. You made me feel that what I have to say is important and warranted all those hours of fine-tuning. My dear sister Rita spent endless hours proofreading the text, correcting my punctuation and making sure my message was coming through clear and true.

I am grateful for all that has happened in the last two and a half years of my life enabling this book to be born: the jolt of losing a dear friend and former client, the solitude provided by being isolated in my home because of the pandemic and the realization that the time had come to let the stories be told.

I am grateful to Avner my husband and partner who was by my side throughout the process. He helped me in subtle yet powerful ways, by believing in me and checking in on me every once in a while to see if I was still breathing.

But, above and beyond all this, I am deeply grateful to all the women who put themselves in my hands and trusted me to be their midwife. I have become who I am today because of you. You enabled me to learn midwifery by doing it, by listening to your fears and concerns, by seeing you sweat and shout and by witnessing your victories.

I see those of you who agreed to have your stories told as co-authors of this book. Working with you allowed me to relive the thrill of each birth. You motivated me to be as accurate as possible in describing the details of your births, from both your perspective and mine. Every story and every one of you has made this path so much more rewarding than I could have ever imagined. I thank you all so much.

References

Balaskas, Janet (1992) *Active Birth: The New Approach to Giving Birth Naturally*, Harvard Common Press.
Bohjalian, Chris (1998) *Midwives*, U.S.A.: Vintage Press.
Charles Smith, Margaret & Holmes, Linda Janet (1996) *Listen to Me Good: The Life Story of an Alabama Midwife*, Ohio State University Press.
Frye, Anne (1997) *Understanding Diagnostic Tests in the Childbearing Year: A Holistic Guide to Evaluating the Health of Mother and Baby*, Oregon, U.S.A.: Labrys Press.
Gaskin, Ina May (1977) *Spiritual Midwifery*, Summertown, TN: Book Pub. Co.
Levine, Peter & Frederick, Ann (1997) *Waking the Tiger*, U.S.A.: North Atlantic Books.
Mongan, Marie F. (2016) *Hypnobirthing: The Mongan Method the Natural Approach to a Safe, Easier, More Comfortable Birthing*, U.S.A.: Health Communications.
Simkin, Penny & Klaus, Phyllis (2004) *When Survivors Give Birth: Understanding and Healing the Effects of Early Sexual Abuse on Childbearing Women*, U.S.A: Quality Code Publishing.
Wainer Cohen, Nancy & Estner, Lois (1983) *Silent Knife – Cesarean Prevention and Vaginal Birth after Cesarean (VBAC)*, U.S.A.: Praeger Publishers Inc.

Wellish, Pam & Root, Susan (1987) *Hearts Open Wide: Midwives & Births*, U.S.A.: Wingbow Press.
https://www.facebook.com/mindy.levy.56/posts/10202860012688960
Levy, Mindy (2004) *Maternity in the Wake of Terrorism: Rebirth or Retraumatization*, Lesley University Graduate School
Levy, Mindy (2006) *Maternity in the Wake of Terrorism: Rebirth or Retraumatization*, Journal of Prenatal and Perinatal Psychology and Health, 20(3): 221-248.
https://midwiferytoday.com
Diary of an Aliyah-nik (2022). Mehmehs
http://www.mehmehs.com/aliyah
Pascali-Bonaro, Debra (Director). (2008) *Orgasmic Birth: The Best-Kept Secret* [Film].

www.ingramcontent.com/pod-product-compliance
Lightning Source LLC
Chambersburg PA
CBHW050726010526
44107CB00009B/746